"Isa Herrera's book showed me the ⸱ .... r myself and how to get out of pain. Th__ ___ ___ ___ ___ ___ yourself using many different types of techniques and exercises. I even learned how to do my own internal massages which reduced my pain and symptoms dramatically. This book improved my confidence and transformed my life. Today I am pain free. Thank you, Isa."

- Monica B.

"This book that Isa Herrera created saved my life. I had a coccyx injury where I couldn't sit or move without excruciating pain. Then I had to get a surgery that left me in even more pain. Isa's book helped me to understand what was going on with me. I also learned how to get myself out of pain and how to avoid extra pain. Isa's book and courses are hands-on, and you will learn different exercises, massages and tools to get yourself better. I highly recommend this book and her programs to any woman who suffers from pelvic floor dysfunction and wants to be able to take care of herself and get rid of her own female symptoms."

- Maria C.

"I felt defeated. I felt overwhelmed, and I believed that life as I knew it had come to a crashing halt. I was able to use this to learn how to treat myself at my own speed and where I was most comfortable. It even enabled me to include my husband in the at-home treatments so that we could work as a team to help keep my conditions in check. After putting in tons of hard work with tons of practice in completing this program, I'm now able to work out again or sit through a movie and have successful sex with my husband, continue to hold down my full-time job, and on a good day, which are more good than bad, I'm even lucky enough to pull off the underwear and jeans thing."

- Tali S.

"I suffered from bladder, vaginal and general pelvic pain for years. All the tools were right there for me in this book. I just had to commit to doing the work and believe that I was going to get better. I can really enjoy my life now. There were points where I thought I would suffer with these symptoms for the rest of my life, and I can finally feel like I'm out of pain, like it's not the everyday nuisance that it once was. I really enjoy my life. I don't feel that I'm inhibited by pain and dysfunction anymore. Really take on this program. Believe in yourself. I know you can get better just like I did."

- Kathleen M.

ISBN: 978-1-946978-15-8

Medical Disclaimer

Consult and seek the advice of your doctor and/or physical therapist before attempting the exercises or self-help tools found in *Female Pelvic Alchemy*. The medical information in this book is provided for informational purposes only, and is not to be used or relied on for any diagnostic or treatment purposes. This information is intended to be educational only and does not create any patient-physical therapist relationship, and should not be used as a substitute for professional diagnosis and treatment. Serious injury could result from improper performance of these techniques and exercises. If pain occurs with any exercise, STOP immediately. Neither *PelvicPainRelief.com* nor Isa Herrera, MSPT, CSCS, can be held liable for injury caused by the improper performance of these exercises or self-help tools. The self-help tips found in this book are merely a guide; this book is not intended as a prescription for physical therapy. To prevent injury seek the advice of your doctor or physical therapist before attempting any exercise, self-help tip or implementation of any of the information in this book. Most patients need a multi-layered approach to overcome their pelvic conditions. Make sure to see doctors and specialists in the field of female gynecology and pelvic floor muscle dysfunction, and then talk to your doctor about getting a referral to a physical therapist that specializes in pelvic floor muscle dysfunction. It is also extremely important to educate yourself about your pelvic condition. Do not be afraid to ask questions of your caregivers, or to get a second opinion about your condition.

For more information about The Female Pelvic Alchemy Online Companion Course, visit:
http://www.PelvicPainRelief.com/FemalePelvicAlchemy

Female Pelvic

Alchemy™

Trade Secrets For Energizing Your Love Life,
Enhancing Your Pleasure &
Loving Your Body Completely

ISA HERRERA
MSPT, CSCS

Dedications

For my husband, David, and daughter, Ella.
Without your endless support and love I could not do what I do.
I love you both very much.
THANK you for everything that you do that keeps us solid as a family.
My heart is full because of the two of you.
You make me want to be a better human.

For Stuart Black,
Who helped awaken me.
You taught me how to search for the truth
with love, compassion, and forgiveness.
I will always be grateful to you.

For my female patients,
You motivate me to think outside the box
to fine-tune the tools and mind-body techniques in this book.
Your stories and firm resolve to end
your dysfunction and pain continue
to fuel my search for answers and to find more
creative ways to help you.

Acknowledgements

David Ondrick, Digital Production, Project Management and Editing
A big heartfelt thanks for your vision. You are an extraordinary man who does what needs to be done without hesitation and with vigor and determination. You are a technical genius and a great friend and husband.

Ella Ondrick, My Loving and Patient Daughter
We are beyond grateful to have your loving energy in our lives. Your patience and understanding during the creative process and production is well beyond your years. We are in awe of your beauty and grace.

Marissa Klapwald, Editor
You have been a light for me. I could not do what I do without your support and guidance. You are a true goddess.

Nancie Salicrup, Makeup Artist
You are a make-up artist extraordinaire!

Richard Simpson, Photographer
Thank you for taking the photos. You always astonish me. You are one creative soul.

Dr. Jacques Moritz, Associate Professor of Obstetrics & Gynecology, Cornell University and Columbia Presbyterian Hospital
Your dedication to the work of helping women always amazes me. I am grateful for your support.

Collin Pisarra & Winston Johnson, Digital Photos and Illustrations. Thank you for being flexible and getting the work done. Your easy nature makes working with you guys a joy.

Crucita Soto, My Mom
You taught me well. You are generous, kind and soulful. You support my family in ways that allow me to do the work that has chosen me.

Adolfo Qanchi Ttito Kuntor, My Mentor
Thank you so much for teaching me the inner workings of the Andean cosmology and for helping me to bring these teachings to my pelvic tribe.

For My Queens

The journey can be long.
It can be hard. It can be good also and amazing.
Life may require that you go where you haven't been before.
You will be tested in ways that can bring you to your knees, but could
lead to more goodness.
You will survive.
Know you are strong.
Know you are enough.
Listen to your heart when it talks to you,
May this book awaken the inner goddess within you
putting you on the road to a more dynamic, more connected, and
healthier you.
Remember your choices today create your destiny tomorrow for
nothing is written in stone and your own healing is within your grasp.
You are your healer. You carry the beacon of light within you.
Reach for it with all your might and don't let go.
It is my hope that this book sheds light on your journey
so your heart can sing and be as free
as the singing **Blue Jay** perched on the tree.

Become the heroine of your own story.™

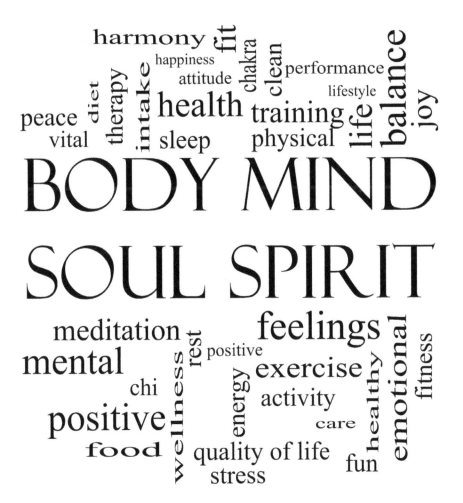

The ABC's Of My "Queendom"

The Queen that lives in you has a message she wants you to know:

- Acknowledge and know that you are gifted, talented and fabulous.
- Blush with me and enjoy those secret moments with me.
- Comfort me and have compassion for me.
- Don't judge me. Love me as I am.
- Energize me.
- Feel the rain, wind, sun and earth with me.
- Grow with me and see me as I am.
- Hug me tightly because I need your love.
- Inspiration is all around you. Seek it. Be your own inspiration.
- Journey with me and explore your body's delights.
- Kink it up with me and dare to be the creatrix of your pleasure.
- Love me dearly and unconditionally.
- Music lives within me so dance with me in the moonlight.
- No is No and Yes is Yes.
- Orgasm with me.
- Power me up when I need it.
- Queen me up and know that you are enough.
- Rejuvenate with me and know that you can reinvent yourself.
- Self-love is the key that will open the doors for you.
- Trust me and listen closely to your heart when it speaks to you.
- Understand me even when I mess up and forgive me.
- Vanquish with me and focus on the positive.
- Wish the best for me and always know that I am on your side.
- Xenia is me.
- Yearn for extraordinary and the goodness.
- Zen out with me and let me be open with you.

Contents

CHAPTER 1

Welcome to Your Queendom

If you are reading this book you are looking to be the creatrix of your pleasure and for natural ways to come back home to your true self. Maybe you've been on what I call the "Doctor Road Show" and you still haven't found solutions to your lady part problems. Maybe you feel that you haven't connected to your inner goddess in a long time and that there should be more to the pleasure you are currently experiencing. Maybe you want a real life with great orgasms, real sex and no pelvic floor muscle dysfunction. You don't know how to heal yourself but you are willing to give self-healing a try.

Now you've come across this book and your insides are yelling: "YES! Yes, this is the answer I've been looking for." Here's the thing—this book is not just for any goddess. This book is for those goddesses who are looking deep inside their souls and have an "I Can Do It Mindset." I'll tell you a secret: You—and only you—hold the key to your "Queendom." There is nothing outside of you that can save you. There is no knight on a white horse. Instead: you are the queen on the white horse that's come to save you. You are the "Heroine of Your Own Story." You are the only one that can do this work. I will be here to guide you and to help you along the way. But at the end of the day you are the one in charge.

Know this in your heart: you have the power to heal yourself. All you need to do is to awaken the doctor within and to trust. Maybe you are still thinking: "I need someone external to myself to heal me." But is this really true? Don't feel badly that no one has given you another choice. We have been conditioned to look outside ourselves for womanly healing. Maybe you feel too damaged; maybe you feel like you are not enough; or maybe you have become disillusioned or stressed because you are not getting better. You shouldn't believe these negative thoughts.

Here's another secret: when you are empowered and understand your body; doors that were closed for you will open again. *This is my promise to you: You are the creatrix of your pelvic healing; when you come from a place of deep understanding only then can you reshape your female pelvic health.*

Always remember: You are enough and you are powerful enough to change your body, your pelvic floor muscles and your destiny.

I have an extraordinary program that is customized to assist you in facilitating your own healing. You do it yourself, but not by yourself because I offer videos, coaching, checklists, support and an invitation to a private Facebook community. I encourage you to explore and look at this option that I have made available for you at: **www.pelvicpainrelief.com/femalepelvicalchemy**

You are probably wondering: who is this woman who is willing to help me transform myself into a goddess? Let me tell you about myself....

Everyone always asks me how I got involved in my line of work. Women treat me with curious interest maybe because they feel hope when they see me. When I was three years old I knew I would be a healer, working with women. There never was another choice for me. I grew up in a household with 7 women so I learned a thing or two about sisterhood. My experiences in the last twelve years—first as a fitness instructor and now as a physiotherapist—have shaped my vision of care and empowerment. After helping thousands of women to heal I decided to write this self-help manual. This is no ordinary book: of course, your incontinence, bladder symptoms and sexual function will most definitely improve with the information in this manual. But beyond this, with *Female Pelvic Alchemy* I want to help women reconnect to their true energetic selves. I want them to remember what it feels like to be whole again. Sexy again. Hot again. I want you to understand that you are a dynamic and beautiful being with so much power inside that all you need is to tap into your power and to set an intention to work and reconnect to your Queendom. There isn't one single source out there that addresses pelvic floor muscle dysfunction from a holistic, energetic, and integrated approach. I want to share with you the tools, exercises and techniques that have worked for my patients, and I want you to have the same success. You deserve it. You need it and you cannot deny yourself this reconnection to yourself any longer.

At my healing center, I give the women under my care many different tools, exercises and techniques to use at home, which I collectively call "The Female Pelvic Alchemy Program." Many find complete relief with my treatments and unique protocols; some experience life-changing relief from their pelvic symptoms. Some reconnect to their orgasms and can now express themselves dynamically to their sexual partners.

This new book, *Female Pelvic Alchemy*, is the next step in bringing my message to a wider audience by incorporating all of my experience into an easy-to-read woman's manual.

I've learned that the women who are the most successful in treating their incontinence, prolapse and sexual dysfunction either possess or develop a positive fighting attitude and learn how to take control of their symptoms on their own. Taking control is not easy, but by incorporating the tools in my book you can give yourself the momentum to get the ball rolling.

You can no longer hide behind excuses. You will have to put yourself first on your own list in order to heal yourself. Don't say things like: "I'm too tired tonight to do my self-healing work." Instead, put aside all your doubts and fears, and decide to become your own savior. As my good friend says: "You are the queen of your Queendom." Queens rise; they don't hide. Rise, my queen, rise. The time is now to reshape your destiny and your love life and your relationship to yourself and your body.

I encourage you to be proactive in your own healing journey and to have an open mind as you go through *Female Pelvic Alchemy* (FPA). FPA is comprehensive and will teach you how to do your own internal vaginal massages and how to develop your own vaginal healing program. How cool is that. The book will introduce you to your anatomy, help you to understand your symptoms and familiarize you with the medical conditions that may be contributing to your pain. It will also show you how to design a pelvic strengthening program that not only works but also ensures long-term success. The pelvic floor muscles (PFMs) are a complex basket of muscles and to get them strong again you have to focus on the whole body. FPA shows you how to align your pelvis, which houses your vaginal pelvic floor muscles. (If the pelvis is out of alignment, then your Kegel program will not be as effective.) The chapter on pelvic alignment is super easy to follow so don't be afraid to tackle this part of your healing journey.

Many women have bladder symptoms because the pelvic floor muscles are not functioning properly and are weak. FPA has one of the most comprehensive chapters on how to tame and control your bladder. I call this "taming the shrew" because your bladder can destroy your goddesses. Simply doing Kegels will not stop you from leaking or having pelvic pressure. Doing more Kegels will not guarantee better orgasms. You need a whole-person approach and you have to develop balance. I will guide you through this process as you move from chapter to chapter.

One of my favorite chapters is **The Truth About Training Your Abdominal Muscles.** The abdominal muscles and the PFMs are in synchronization with each other. So if you have a Diastasis Recti Abdominal (DRA) separation or abdominal weakness your PFMs will not get strong no matter how many Kegels you do. You must strengthen both the core and the PFMs at the same time to maximize your pelvic health. This is a unique approach that I have used for almost a decade and it works. I developed my abdominal program after treating hundreds of women crunching themselves into dysfunction and organ prolapse. You need a strong core to keep your lady parts in their right places. Don't worry if you've been doing traditional crunches. You will finally get the abdominal power and beauty you have been seeking.

Many women tell me that their orgasms are not what they used to be: they are weak, non-existent or it takes a long time to reach sexual peak. Sexual dysfunction can be a complex issue, but why not address the PFMs, which play a huge part in sexual function and help produce stronger orgasms? FPA has two important chapters that help improve sexual function; these chapters show you sexual healing exercises, chakra balancing exercises and integrative therapies. You will be pleased with the results and you will able to reclaim your sex life with the information in FPA.

I have saved the best for last. I am all about female power. But many times women are either prescribed Kegels incorrectly and/or they are performing way too many creating more sexual problems. Female sexual power is all about balance. If you Kegel, then what happens after that? You need to incorporate the reverse Kegel into every Kegel.

In the Alchemical Kegel chapter you will be blown away by the trade secrets I share with you—information previously known only to women's health experts. You will finally get the scoop on Kegels and their counterpart reverse Kegels. Kegel therapy is an art form. It is not just about excessively contracting "the down-there muscles." FPA shows you what is missing in many of the books written today. I actually coined the term "reverse Kegel" because women got it when I used this phrase. When they understood this delicate balance and got it just right—WOW!—the results were amazing.

FPA has many tools, exercises and techniques; some may work for you and others may cause you pain or increase your pelvic symptoms. You must follow your womanly intuition and inner guide when working with the tools in FPA. If it hurts, stop, reassess and ask yourself if this technique or exercise is the right one for you. Ask: "Am I being too aggressive with the tools? If I do this technique gently and slowly, will it hurt less and give me pain relief?" Oftentimes, the techniques you try will cause some pain as you take back control of your body, but just remember to listen to the messages your body is sending you. This is part of the healing goddess trip. Listening.

Keep track of the tools and exercises that you do and become your own expert on what helps to relieve your pelvic symptoms and connect to your inner sexual being. Understand that when you use the tools in this book you will have setbacks. This is normal. At times, you may experience more symptoms. This is normal. The body has to catch up. The mind has to catch up. Wait a few days and see how you feel. If symptoms flare up due to the exercises, you may feel worse for 24 to 72 hours, but eventually, you will feel better. This is very true when it comes to massaging your vagina. It's the same as when you work out at the gym. There's always muscle soreness.

I have a special treat for you. At the end of each chapter I give you a link where you can get extra informational videos, downloads, and information that will help you go deeper in your healing. All you have to do is go to http://www.femalepelvicalchemy.com to take your healing to an even deeper level.

I have covered the overall background to my mission and have primed you to get started. Remember that ultimately you hold the key to your own healing. You are the emerging goddess. Go through this book carefully and with an open mind.

Your road to healing will require commitment and a readiness to make the following promises:

1. Open-mindedness and a strong intent to do the work that is required of you. You can't succeed and recapture your inner goddess via osmosis. You will become master with practice.

2. Renunciation of negative self-talk, negative thinking and catastrophic thinking. All your thoughts carry energy. Watch how you talk to yourself and be kind and compassionate to yourself.

3. Sacrifice of your time. You will need to work within this program one hour per day initially. Athletes have to train. If you want to return and reconnect with yourself you have to put in the time.

4. You must have an internal desire to get better. The healing process takes time and you may experience setbacks. Why do the program if you feel you can't get better? Thoughts like this are defeatist and counterproductive.

5. A commitment to stay in the present moment without projecting into the future or the past. What's happened has happened. You cannot change that. Self-forgiveness will help you to let go or

simply release all the negativity that you've experienced in your heart, soul and *yoni*. I know this is hard but you can do this.

6. An understanding on your part that there is no cookie-cutter approach to this program. You must experiment with all the tools and discover what exercises or techniques work best for you.

7. Patience with yourself and the ability to learn all the tools in this book. You will need to practice many times to master the techniques and exercises covered here.

8. You must have focused attention when using the tools in this book. If you don't, you risk hurting or injuring yourself. Focus, focus and focus some more.

9. You must listen to your body; never override a pain signal or a voice in your head that tells you something is wrong. It could save you from a flare-up or more pain.

10. Fearlessness. You must be fearless and understand you are not alone. Always remind yourself you are a fearless goddess. Don't let fear stop you from achieving your goals and getting your life back. Your destiny is within your reach.

I have read the above requirements and I understand what it will take to heal. This signature serves as a contract between my inner healer and me. I understand that I alone hold the key to my healing.

Your signature here

Now that you understand what is required of you, read *Female Pelvic Alchemy* and make yourself the heroine of your own story. Welcome to your Queendom.

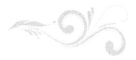

You have come this far, but I have more to teach you.

Welcome to Your Queendom

…to go deeper ONLINE, visit
http://www.FemalePelvicAlchemy.com/chapter1

In this special download I take you deeper into your female healing and give you extraordinary tips on how to supercharge your Female Pelvic Alchemy program to get the best possible results. Here you will find the fountain of youth and fountain of health.

CHAPTER 2

Taking Care of Your Lady Business Naturally

The same old ways of doing things no longer work for most women. Today women are searching for something more. Something magical and different that doesn't require taking a bunch of pills or surrendering their power to someone else. Women with pelvic dysfunction and sexual needs want a fresh perspective when it comes to treating and taking care of themselves. In this chapter I share with you my most tried-and-true integrative therapies that I give women who seek help from me. Alternative healers use much of what is covered in this chapter, and I have also successfully used many of the therapies on many patients. It is my sincere hope that they also bring you relief and results.

We'll start with acupressure therapy. This East-meets-West medicine is an important part of my pelvic alchemy self-care program. I have also included a section on vulvar care and how to do a vulvar exam, because you will be building on this anatomy when it comes to strengthening and creating balance in your PFMs. Most women know that they should examine their breasts on a monthly basis but few know that they should also examine their vulvar area. I want you to be familiar with proper vulvar-vaginal care because many times incorrect vulvar care can be a trigger for female pelvic pain and sexual dysfunction.

I am a certified Mayan abdominal practitioner and as part of this massage I frequently recommend vaginal steams (also known as V-steams). Vaginal steams are very healing for the pelvic muscles and I give you step-by-step information on how to do them in this chapter. I also recommend Castor oil packs for many of my female patients. They help with improving circulation and breaking up abdominal scar tissue—very important for the many women I treat with abdominal scars that impede the function and strength of pelvic floor and abdominal muscles.

This chapter is for every woman who is looking to think outside the box and wants to take charge of her health. These therapies help many of my patients reclaim their female power and sexual sovereignty. Whether you want to stay within the goddess realm or are looking to find your way back home to your inner goddess, this chapter is a must-read.

Wakening and Balancing the Chi with Acupressure Therapy

Acupressure is one of my go-to techniques to help patients stay in prime health. I love it for its effectiveness and simplicity in treating female gynecological problems. I became interested in acupressure points when I accidently found that if I pressed certain spots on the body, the patient would have a tremendous amount of relief not only from physical pain but also from anxiety and stress.

One of the oldest medical systems in existence, acupressure comes from China. It is performed on meridian lines, the pathways or channels in which our energy circulates throughout our bodies. There are 12 meridians plus two special meridians called the Governor Vessel and the Conception Vessel. Associated with organs of the body, meridians are named for the organs they correspond to, the positions they hold, and their yin and yang properties.

The yin meridians are located in the front of the body, while the yang meridians are at the back of the body. The yin and yang are paired meridians; if there's an issue with one, then there's an issue with the other.

The points that are used in traditional acupuncture are also used in acupressure. Because acupressure points are located on meridian lines, these external points allow access to your internal energy. Many points take their names from their positions. For instance, Spleen 6 is located on the spleen meridian and it is the 6th point on that system. Many other points have traditional names.

Acupressure points tend to be sensitive and sometimes painful in those who are compromised. When I press a point the patient can feel energy or pain radiating into the meridian or associated body part. This is a normal response. Patients are often surprised by how painful this therapy can be. When working on yourself, slow, steady and gentle pressure is recommended. Do no put excessive pressure on a point.

Acupressure point therapy can help treat many ailments. It works beautifully to support your healing process and to address energetic disharmony. In the pages that follow, I will discuss the acupressure points that I have found to be clinically relevant to issues related to female health and emotional balance.

Keep these things in mind before you begin your own acupressure point therapy program:

1. When there's a medical issue involved, my recommendation is that you first see your doctor.

2. If you are unsure how to proceed with point therapy, go to an acupuncturist who can review and teach you the points.

3. I recommend you massage acupressure points in a clockwise direction for 1 to 2 minutes or apply direct pressure for 1 to 2 minutes.

4. You may feel a slight pulsation at the points when you work on them. This is a good sign that the circulation has improved and that the point has been activated.

5. Point therapy can be done daily or every other day depending on how your body responds.

6. Listen closely to your body and do not address too many points at once. I would keep the acupressure treatment to 3 to 5 points.

Be sure to review and observe the sensible precautions and guidelines described in Table 2.1 so that you can apply acupressure to yourself safely.

Table 2.1 Precautions When Using Acupressure Point Therapy

Avoid Acupressure Point Therapy with:
• **Pregnancy:** there are many points that you should not press during pregnancy because doing so can cause uterine contractions. If you are pregnant, consult with a professional acupuncturist before trying any of the points listed in this chapter.
• Acute Infection of any kind.

• Issues with the spine such as herniated disc or slipped disc.
• Heart attacks.
• Circulation problems.
• Issues with bone health such as osteoporosis.
• Illnesses such as colds, flus, high fevers.
• Issues with arteries or problems with blot clotting and/or blood thinning medications.
• Cancer, epilepsy.
• Pain that is strong.
• Uncertainty: **Don't guess;** if you are unsure of the point you are on, don't do the acupressure therapy.
• Recent surgery: get medical clearance before you press the points covered in this chapter.
• Acute muscle, bone or tendon injury. This can cause serious damage.
• Scars that have not healed.

How to Apply Pressure to an Acupressure Point

This type of therapy requires that you stay in the present moment and are tranquil. Start in a quiet room, making sure you are as relaxed and as comfortable as possible. Focus on your breathing; the breath should be slow and steady.

I use two types of pressure: **steady pressure** and **circulating pressure.** Begin by applying pressure to the point using one or two fingertips. The fingers should be bent and perpendicular to the point. Once your fingers are in this position, apply **gentle steady pressure.**

It can be painful or you may experience a stabbing needle-like feeling. If you start to get tense you are applying too much pressure. Release the pressure so that it's effective but not so painful that you are contracting your body. Once you find your perfect pressure you can just hold the point steady or perform **gentle circular massage** on the point. If you want to increase the pressure on the point it is best to do so while exhaling. When rubbing or massaging a point use pressure that is comfortable and stimulating.

Breathing and Acupressure Therapy

Breath work plays an important role while pressing a point; for best results you should coordinate your breathing with the acupressure pressing. Start by exhaling and pressing on the point. Hold for several breathing cycles. When you are ready to release the point, inhale. When you release the pressure, do so slowly as you inhale. As far as how long to hold it: you will know when it feels right to release. (As a general guideline: up to 2 minutes and 2 to 3 cycles on each point.) Many times when I am working on a chronic patient I press for 30 seconds and do 1 to 3 cycles.

Table 2.2 lists my best acupressure points, the points I use on myself and on my patients. Over the years I have found these to be the most beneficial and I consider them to be an important part of a goddess's self-care program. For each point on the list, I will explain how to find the point, how to perform acupressure on the point, and what benefit you can expect to derive from the therapy.

Table 2.2 Acupressure Points in the Goddess Self-Care Program

• Spleen 6
• Sacrum Massage for Female Wellness
• Open the Heart Goddess Point: Shen Men
• Large Intestine 4: Take My Pain Away
• Conception Vessel (Ren Channel) Ren Three
• Hui Yin Point (Ren 1) at the First Chakra (Perineum)
• Ren Points Massage for Bladder, Sex, Menstrual and Other Female Issues
• Bai Hui Point AKA Hundred Converges Point
• Yin Tang Point
• Leg Three Miles (Stomach 36)

Spleen 6

I use this point frequently in connection with female gynecological issues.

How to Find: Find the inner part of your ankle and place your four fingers at the top of the ankle bone. The point is located here on the back edge of the shin. It can be very painful and many of my pelvic patients complain about deep pain when I use it. Sometimes they tell me they feel lighter in the pelvis. It's always a good idea to warm up a point by rubbing the ankle. *This point is not to be used in pregnancy because it can increase contractions.*

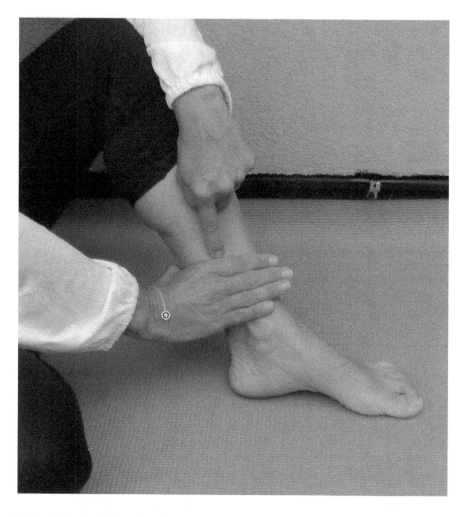

Why It's Goddess Medicine: Relieves menstrual cramps, urological issues, pelvic congestion and insomnia.

Sacrum Massage for Female Wellness

How to Find: The sacrum is located in the center of your buttocks. It is a diamond-shaped bone that houses many muscles, ligaments and nerves. It also houses the Urinary Bladder points 27 through 35. To work these points we will use massage.

Lie on your side and massage your sacrum back and forth for up to 5 minutes until you feel the sacrum warm up. Make sure to massage and rub the whole sacrum. *Do not massage these points in pregnancy. This could cause uterine contractions.*

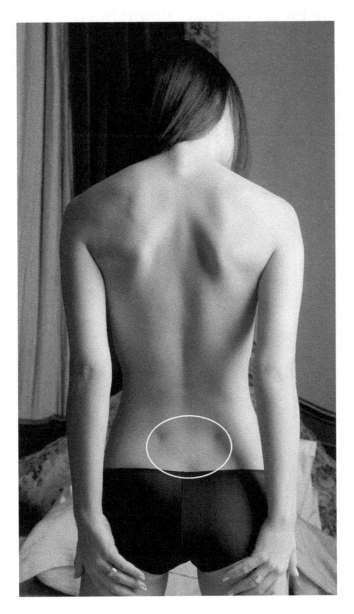

Why It's Goddess Medicine: These points help to treat problems with the lower body, gynecological problems related to menstruation, sacral pain, sciatic pain and hemorrhoids.

Open the Heart Goddess Point: Shen Men

This is one of my favorite points; I use it all the time on my patients and myself. It is called the Shen Men point or the Spirit Gate. Massaging or pressing this point helps to reduce anxiety and stress and connects us to our celestial energy. This point is a heart point and it is believed that when you press this point you connect your voice to your heart and to a higher spirit. Shen Men promotes tranquility and harmony.

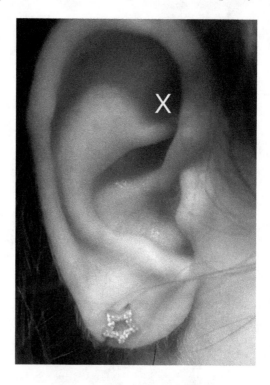

How to Find: Locate the outer part of the ear and you will find a ridge. That ridge subdivides into two ridges creating an indentation or gully. Place your finger inside the gully and your thumb on the back of the ear and press the two together.

Why It's Goddess Medicine: This point helps to alleviate stress, pain, tension, anxiety, depression and insomnia. The ultimate goddess point, Shen Men promotes harmony, connection and tranquility.

Large Intestine 4: Take My Pain Away

How to Find: This point is in the top of the hand between the first and second metacarpal bones or the place where your index finger bone and your thumb bone meet. It's the web space between your thumb and index finger.

Why It's Goddess Medicine: This point helps to relieve pain related to muscles, bones and/or headaches.

Conception Vessel (Ren Channel) Ren Three

How to Find: This channel runs down the front middle line of your body. It is sometimes referred to as the Functional Channel. This amazing point is located approximately four inches below the navel

Why It's Goddess Medicine:
This point helps with:

- strengthening the kidneys, improving the genitals and regulating menstruation
- relieving pelvic pain and boosting the libido
- strengthening the urinary and reproductive system
- increasing sexual pleasure. Great for all female problems and super sexy if your partner massages it for you.

Hui Yin Point (Ren 1) at the First Chakra (Perineum)

How to Find: This point is located between the anus and the vagina. It is called the central tendon, the perineum or perineal body. I like to call it the Queen's Castle. I use it to energize myself and my patients' sexual energy. I also use it as part of my program with women who suffer from pelvic pain. Several of the pelvic floor muscles converge here, so it's truly a point that improves sexual power and helps to restore flexibility and suppleness to the pelvic floor muscles. (Later on, I'll discuss anatomy to give you a deeper understanding of this point's importance to women's sexuality and pelvic health.) Many women experience perineal tears or episiotomies during childbirth or as a result of surgeries, and these tears can compromise the function of this point. With a deep connection to our energy and pelvic floor muscles, this point also connects the Conception and Governor channels so it is important that we keep it healthy and flexible. Place your finger at the point and do small circular massages.

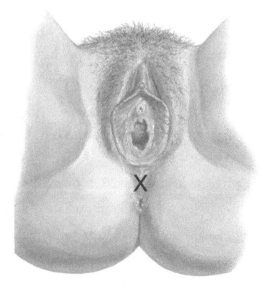

Source: Netter Images.

Why It's Goddess Medicine: Contracting this point allows energy to flow up through the spine. This point also helps to:

- generate and flow more sexual energy throughout the body and to increase vitality to the vagina
- hold our organs in place (it is considered to be the primary support for our organs)
- relieve pelvic congestion.

Ren Points Massage for Bladder, Sex, Menstrual and Other Female Issues

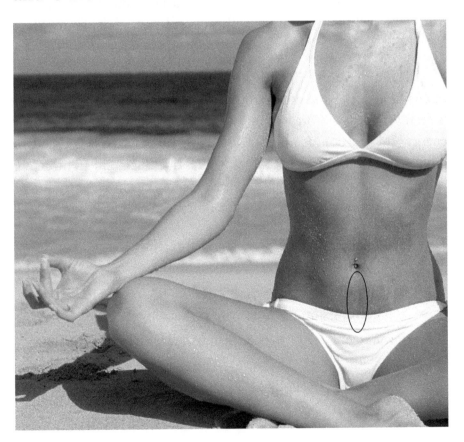

How to Find: These points are part of the Conception Vessel channel. There are 24 points in all on this channel. The lower abdomen (below the abdomen) contains 7 acupressure points with the first point on the perineum (which we discussed above). All the points are found at the midline of the body so they are easy to find. For bladder issues you can work the points below the navel. Start below the navel at the center of the body. Massage this point for ten seconds and then go to the point below it. Continue in this manner until you reach the edge of the pubic bone. Before going to the next point do about 5 to 10 gentle downward strokes toward the pubic bone. (The sequence is: massage the point for 1 to 2 minutes and then perform gentle downward strokes toward the pubic bone. Proceed to the next point.) There are about 7 points in this below-the-belly-button midline. They are all part of the Conception Vessel and are called Ren points. *Not to be used in pregnancy.*

A special note on Ren Three: This point is located 4 fingers below the navel at the center of the body. It is sometimes call the "O" point meaning this is the orgasm point. This point helps improve sexual energy and function. It's been said that if you massage and tune this point up you can achieve an orgasm. Massage this point right before you plan to make love for up to 2 minutes in a clockwise direction or do a sustained hold. This point is one of my personal favorites.

Why It's Goddess Medicine:
These points help with:

- urinary tract infections
- regulating lower abdominal functionality
- improving fertility, incontinence, menstrual irregularities, and low libido
- improving, strengthening and facilitating orgasms.

Bai Hui Point AKA Hundred Converges Point

How to Find: The Bai Hui point is the uppermost point of the body located at the top of the crown. This is a master point said to treat 100 ailments. At the Bai Hui point there is a convergence of the six yang channels and the Governing vessel. Its power should not be underestimated. Place the tips of your thumbs at the uppermost point of your ears and then reach your middle fingers across your head so they touch one another, at the crown of your head. When I get my acupuncture treatments I always ask for an acupuncture needle at this point. I love to use this point when I need to be more connected to a person or when I am being creative (such as writing a book). I feel that this point opens me up while grounding me at the same time. It helps improve my Queendom and my intuition. *Do not use in pregnancy.*

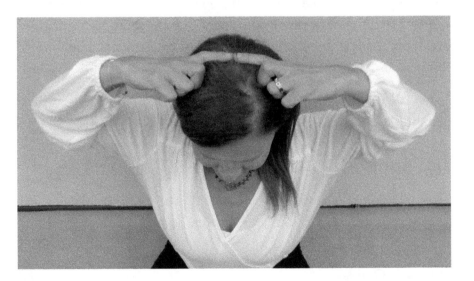

Why It's Goddess Medicine:
This point helps with:

- relieving headaches and prolapse of the uterus or rectum
- clearing the head and calming the spirit
- experiencing duress or anxiety
- promoting relaxation and mental clarity at the same time
- chronic fatigue
- improving intuition and connection.

Yin Tang Point

How to Find: This is another favorite. It's called an extraordinary point and I feel that to be true. This point is located between the eyebrows at center of the forehead where you would find the location of the third eye. It can be massaged either clockwise or counterclockwise for 1 to 2 minutes.

Why It's Goddess Medicine: This point helps to relieve anxiety, agitation or insomnia.

Leg Three Miles (Stomach 36)

How to Find: Located on the front of the leg four fingers below the kneecap, on the outside, in the depression between the shin bone and the anterior tibialis leg muscle.

Why It's Goddess Medicine: Stomach 36 increases stamina and energy and provides a sense of overall well being. It heals the body when you are worried or overthinking a situation and reduces anxiety. Do not abuse this point to give yourself energy when you are exhausted; it will backfire. Use once a week.

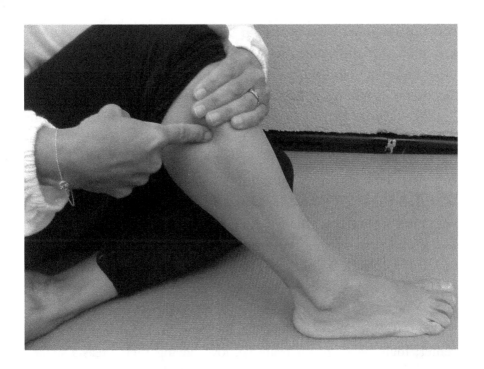

Getting to Know Yourself:
How to Perform a Self-Examination of the
Vulvar-Vaginal Area

You've tried acupressure therapy—what's next? You cannot be successful with your own self-care unless you take the time to examine yourself and learn to understand the uniqueness of your Queendom. Many of the women I treat start out in my healing center completely disconnected to their pelvic floor muscles and vaginas. I tell them that they have to change this outlook in order to have any chance at successfully recapturing their inner goddess. Get to know your body first so you can get on the road to recovery and long-lasting results.

I also have treated many women who tell me they hate their vaginas, and I find that statement very disheartening. Your vagina is beautiful. It is your Queendom and the center of immense pleasure. Your vagina contains the inner parts of the clitoris and has deep erogenous tissue inside of it. Many women have vaginal orgasms via the G-spot and other orgasms from having just fingers inside of them or from having a penis go in and out of the vagina.

My favorite female organ is the clitoris. The clitoris is the only organ in our bodies whose sole function is PLEASURE. It contains 8,000 nerve ending. When you are using the mirror to explore your lady parts look at your vagina with new eyes. Focus on all the beauty of it. Tell yourself: "I love you so much. Thank you for providing me with pleasure and life." The self-examination allows you to explore and feel which parts of your vulva light you up and make you delicious inside and outside. It's not purely a medical process but an exploration of your Queendom. I have seen over 14,000 vaginas and no two look alike. Your vulva, vagina, and clitoris are unique to you. How wonderful is that. They make up your pleasure center. But this is not the *only* center; many women, for example, love having their breasts sucked or massaged. We are traditionally told to do breast exams to screen for cancer but are not told to explore our breast for pleasure. I believe that this is a monthly exercise that needs to be incorporated into the Emerging Goddess's self-care program. Make sure to look at and touch all the different parts of the vulvar-vaginal area. Keep a diary with your results. What have you discovered? What turns you on? What is your relationship with her and how can you improve it? How will you communicate with your partner on how you like to be touched?

Now let's take a look at the Queendom and let's explore. Only say nice things to her. If you find yourself judging her, change that thought immediately. Remember that we are not our thoughts; we are so much better than the voice in our heads. Your inner critic must not win her. This is an exploration of love. At the end of your exploration don't forget to rub her nicely and gently. Send love into your lady parts and see how it changes your relationship with her.

Make sure to perform your exam in a well-lit place. You will also need a mirror, Q-tip and lubricant. There are many positions in which you can perform your vulvar examination. Find a position that you are comfortable in that allows you to examine the whole area. Recommended positions for this examination are: sitting with legs apart, standing with one leg up or squatting over a mirror. Hold your mirror up close to examine all the external parts. To examine the inner parts you will have to spread your vaginal lips to expose the vulvar area.

Checking All of Your Queendom

The vulva is made up of the following structures: labia majora, labia minora, clitoris, vestibule of the vagina, bulb of the vestibule, and the glands of Bartholin. We will also examine the perineum in addition to the vulva.

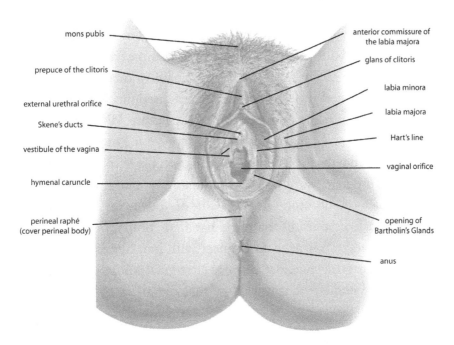

mons pubis

anterior commissure of
the labia majora

prepuce of the clitoris

glans of clitoris

labia minora

external urethral orifice

labia majora

Skene's ducts

Hart's line

vestibule of the vagina

hymenal caruncle

vaginal orifice

perineal raphé
(cover perineal body)

opening of
Bartholin's Glands

anus

External Genitalia, Part of Layer 1 of the Pelvic Floor Muscles. Source: Netter Images.

Check Your Mons Pubis

This is the area where your pubic hair and pubic bone are located. Sometimes this is an area of pain for women who have bladder conditions. This is sometimes called the mons of Venus. Many women no longer have pubic hair in this area. Softly explore your Venus and massage it. Does it turn you on? The nerve to the clitoris has a deep relationship here. Many women use their vibrators to the side of the Venus mons because they can get access to the nerve to clitoris here.

What to Look For: Run your fingers along the skin and feel for any bumps, warts, or sores. Also examine the area for any color changes in the skin such as red, white or dark spots. Look for pleasure spots along the mons. What did you find?

Check Your Clitoris

Feel and look at your clitoris and the surrounding area. Also gently pull back on the hood of the clitoris. My favorite lady part is the clitoris, the only organ made solely for our pleasure. Some women can only have clitoral orgasms and others find themselves disconnected due to pain here. There is a fine line between pain and pleasure. We have to make sure that it's moving well, and below I show you how to make sure the clitoris is moving freely in its hood. If you are using a vibrator on the clitoris, use a gentle speed. I've had many women hurt the clitoris from overusing a vibrator. Use the palm of your hand to massage it. How do you like your clitoris to be handled? Softly, fast, or pitched between fingers? You need to connect with her. She is here to give you earth-shattering pleasure but you first must know how she likes to be handled and in what way. Note that the gland of the clitoris is the external part of the clitoris but much of it lies inside the body. It is designed this way so that this precious organ is protected inside of our bodies.

What to Look For: Does the clitoral hood move or is it bound down? The clitoris should freely move in its hood. Also examine the clitoris for coloring, pain and inflammation by lightly touching it with your finger or Q-tip.

If you find that the clitoris is not moving freely add the next technique to your Emerging Goddess self-care program.

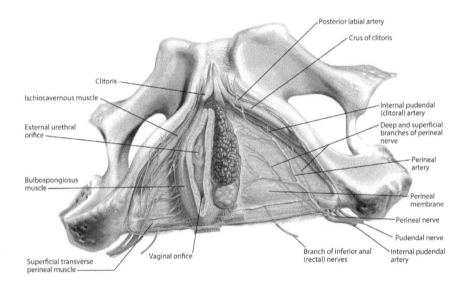

Source: Netter Images.

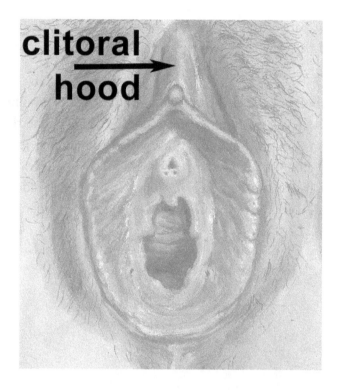

Source: Netter Images

The clitoral hood protects the clitoral gland and should move freely. Sometimes women experience adhesions of the clitoral hood and the hood can get bound down. This lack of movement can be a major cause of clitoral pain and decreased sensation. The gentle technique described below is very effective and will help you to reach new heights of pleasure. I call it the Clitoral Hood Release and Stretch. We release and then stretch to feel more pleasure.

Clitoral Hood Release and Stretch Overview

WHAT TO DO:

Locate your clitoris by following your labia minora upward until you have located the glans of the clitoris (external part). The hood covers the glans clitoris. Imagine the top part of the hood as a clock. Twelve o'clock is at the middle, 1 o'clock to the left and 11 o'clock to the right. Gently place your index finger at the12 o'clock position and gently move the hood slightly upward. Hold for 3 to 5 seconds or as tolerated. Now repeat the same process at the 11 o'clock and 1 o'clock positions. Repeat two to three times at each clock point. Monitor for pain and avoid pain levels over three. Use a mirror to see where the clitoral hood is moving or not moving and so that you can track your progress.

Clitoral Hood Stretch

WHAT TO DO:
Once the hood is freed up and moving well you can start to incorporate the clitoral hood stretching. Locate your clitoris by following your labia minora upward until you have located the glans of the clitoris (external part). Place your index finger at the 12 o'clock position above the glans but on the superior part of the clitoral hood. Place the other index finger on the upper part of the labia minora but below the glans clitoris. Maintaining a firm sustained pressure on the labia minora pull the hood gently upward toward the pubic bone until you feel a gentle stretch. Hold for up to 10 seconds or as tolerated. Repeat 2 to 3 times.

Check Your Labia Minora and Feel for Pleasure

The vaginal lips get more commentary from women than any other lady parts. I hear it all: "My lips are too small," "My lips are too big," "My lips are not even," "My lips are not open enough," and so forth and so on. Ladies, our lips are the landing places for our pleasure. We have way too much judgment on them. Many women tell me that they like their vaginal lips to be sucked or licked during sex. This opened my eyes. It's not all about the clitoris. The lips are also part of our delicious Queendom and deserve respect, love and less negativity. We have been conditioned by porn and other sex magazines that our vaginas and lips need to look a certain way. But no, they don't need to look a certain way. The universe gave you your perfect vaginal lips and we have to turn this judgment into an act of self-love for our sake and survival. Let's take a look at our inner lips now; these are located to the right and left of the vaginal opening.

What to Look For: Look and touch by holding the labial skin between thumb and fingers. Check on all sides of the labia – front and back and both sides, right and left. Run your fingers along the skin and feel for what brings you pleasure. Of course, we must also look on the medical side of things especially if we are sexually active. After your pleasure exploration look for any bumps, warts, or sores. Examine the area for any color changes in the skin such as red, white or dark spots. Look for ulcers, sores, small blisters, and areas of pain, swelling and inflammation. This area can appear very red and inflamed in women with pelvic floor dysfunction and in women suffering from vulvar vestibulitis or vestibulodynia. Keep in mind that the inner lips are not always pink; their coloring is unique to you and can range from pink to deep pink to dark brown. So don't believe all those airbrushed pictures of vaginas that you see in magazines.

Check Your Labia Majora and Talk Right to Her

Here is another hot topic: I see women getting vaginoplasty surgeries because they simply cannot stand the way their large lips look. I hold no judgment. But these surgeries are serious business and come with a slew of complications including pain and scar tissue. After these surgeries, many women experience pain with sex and their pelvic floor muscles are hypertonic meaning they are too tight and can't relax.

Our womanly health relies on supple, flexible and balanced pelvic floor muscles. Wouldn't it be easier if we tried to have a more loving compassionate relationship with our genitalia? Wouldn't it be easier if we could stop talking negatively to our vaginas? Imagine your friend came to you and asked: "Hey, what do you think about my vagina?" What would you tell her? I am sure you would be kind and say that her vagina is beautiful and perfect the way it is. Use that analogy and think about the way you are talking to "her"—is it with loving kindness? These are your outer vaginal lips next to the labia minora. Slide your fingers along the outer lips, both sides. Many of my patients have labial pain, trigger points or itching along the length of the outer labia. Massage and cross friction massage work great in reducing pain in this area.

What to Look For: Look for pleasure; look for pain, look for restrictions. Remember that the outer vaginal lips have a relationship with the pelvic floor muscles especially the first layer, the sexual layer. Many times pain with sex can be remedied by treating the outer vaginal lips. Also note that the pudendal nerve, which gives us orgasms and sexual powers also has nerve endings on the large vaginal lips. Keeping the lips supple and pain-free adds to your sexual power and strength of orgasms. Roll the lips, massage the lips and see if you find a painful area. Do a pain-release technique by holding the spot gently for 90 seconds or until the pain subsides.

Labia Stretch, Roll and Cross Friction Massage

The labia are truly amazing female structures that provide us with access to nerves, muscles, and erectile tissue. This type of stretching and mobilization is great for women who are having pain with initial penetration or for women whose pelvic floor muscles are too tight and painful for intercourse. Working on the labia will also help women suffering from pudendal nerve neuralgia. When performing these techniques, focus on increasing the flexibility and suppleness of the labial tissue. These techniques are also great to use when you have your period and do not want to do internal vaginal work.

Labia Stretch

WHAT TO DO:

Anchor your finger on the top of the right labia majora near the clitoris. Place the thumb of the opposite hand at the bottom of the same labia and stretch downward. Hold for 30 seconds to 1 minute, repeating 2 to 3 times and then switch to the other labia.

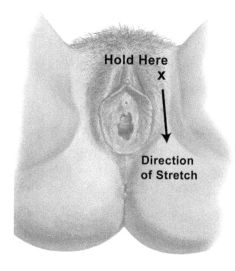

Base Image Source: Netter Images

Labia Roll (no illustration)

Pinch the right labia majora between the thumb and the forefinger. Roll the tissue gently between the fingers until you reach the bottom.

You can roll the labia tissue in either an upward or downward direction; choose the direction that is least painful for you. Repeat 2 to 3 times and then switch sides. Be very gentle and soft when working on this delicate structure.

Labia Cross Friction Massage

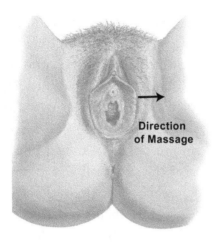

Direction of Massage

Base Image Source: Netter Images.

Place your index or forefinger on the top of your right labia majora. Gently massage the tissue across the labia from side to side until you reach the bottom. Repeat 2 to 3 times and then switch sides. *To create a loving relationship with your outer vaginal lips, speak kindly to them when performing the above techniques. Treat them well and they will be kind to you in return.*

The Seat of Our Queendom: Hui Yin Point (Ren 1)

Although the perineum and the vestibule (the area that surrounds your vaginal opening) are typically not included in the vulvar self-examination, I highly recommend that you do not overlook them in your monthly Emerging Goddess self-care examination. Examining these areas will give you tremendous insight into your pelvic pain condition.

The Seat of Your Queendom also known in medical terms as the perineum is the area between your vagina and anus. This is where doctors perform an episiotomy, which is a surgical cut of the perineum done just before the delivery of a child. Many women who experience pain have scar tissue in this area as a result of an episiotomy or surgery. This area is a highway for many muscles and it provides us with an external view of the levator ani muscles, also known as pelvic floor muscles. Palpation or touching of this area will give you an idea about what is going on internally in your pelvic floor muscles such as flexibility, mobility and pain and whether there's too much laxity in the pelvic floor muscles. If there's too much tone in this area, then there's an added risk for pelvic floor dysfunction such as pain, weakness or sexual issues. If there's too little tone, then there's a risk for pelvic floor muscle dysfunction that can contribute to organ prolapse, incontinence, and/ or weak orgasms. We want this area to have a balanced tone: not too much and not too little.

What to Look For: First, look for scar tissue, lesions, and sores. Also examine the area for any color changes in the skin such as red, white or dark spots. Many times this area becomes red and hyper-irritable due to the dysfunction that is present in the pelvic floor muscles. When the muscles of the vagina function better, the redness and irritation in this area disappears. You will need a mirror and to be in a well-lit room for this exam as well.

Now look at the perineal body. This is the midpoint of the perineum. Testing this area for mobility and ease of movement will give you an insight as to what is going on in your pelvic muscles. When you are performing a Kegel correctly this area moves up toward your head and in toward your body. When performing a reverse Kegel—a relaxation Kegel—the seat moves toward the feet. It is important to incorporate both a Kegel and reverse Kegel into your Emerging Goddess Program. (Following this brief introduction, I cover how to create your own goddess program in the chapters that follow.)

In a reverse Kegel the perineum, "the seat of your Queendom," should drop down or come forward toward your mirror. When you do a Kegel this is the area that you want to see move up toward your head. If there's tightness here or too much flexibility you will have some difficulty in improving your sexual power and orgasms. There are several techniques that will help you to get rid of pain or tightness in this area and that will also improve your orgasms and overall function.

Pressing into the Queendom Seat

In some pelvic surgeries and during childbirth this area can get traumatized. The site where episiotomies are frequently performed, this is a big source of pain for new moms who have experienced a perineal tear. Many times you can relieve pelvic pain by working and finding trigger points in this area. If you've had a surgery you will need to get medical clearance before doing this technique.

WHAT TO DO:

1. Start your investigation by pressing along the perineal area. Take note of where the pain is and what symptoms you feel when you press into these areas.

2. Make yourself a simple map. Note pain level from 0 to 10 (0 = no pain, 10 = worst pain) and symptoms produced. Think of the perineum as a clock as you did with other techniques.

3. For best results, try pressing into the perineal body at different angles and locations in the perineum. Hold each different direction for up to 90 seconds or as tolerated. The goal is to promote flexibility and to decrease pain and/or symptoms by 50 percent.

Location of the Queendom Seat

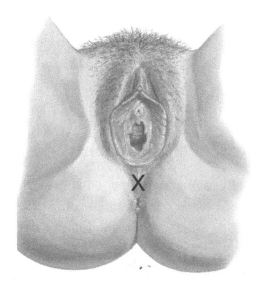

Base Image Source: Netter Images.

Many times I will instruct my patients to gently move this area to the left, right, up, and down and to feel in which direction it is not moving freely. Once you have established that, stretch the perineal body into that direction by holding it in the stretch position for 30 seconds to one minute.

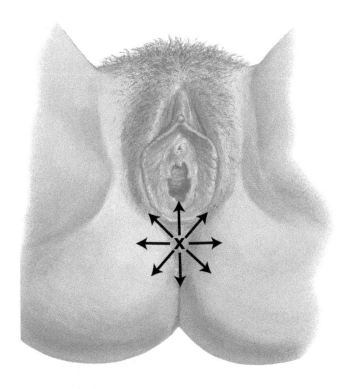

Description: How to find tension in your "Queendom Seat."
Source: Netter Images.

You can also stretch your "Queendom Seat" by gently pressing down on the perineum with one or two thumbs at the 6 o'clock position. Performing this internal stretch helps us to keep our vaginas and pelvic floor muscles flexible, strong and supple. Many women suffer from tight vaginal muscles rather than overstretched vaginal muscles. I also find that there can be a lot of pain in this area that needs to resolve so there's no pain with sex especially initial penetration. This is an amazing vaginal stretch that keeps us fully connected to our inner goddess.

Your Vagina Is a Three-Dimensional Queen

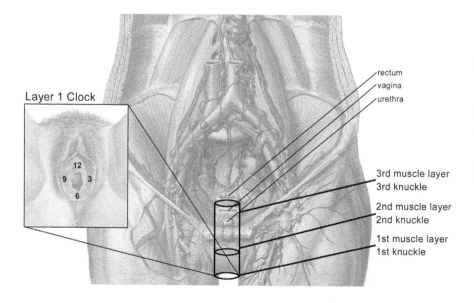

Source: Netter Images.

To visualize the technique, imagine that your vagina is 3-dimensional, like a tube. There are 3 layers to the tube from superficial to the deepest layer. The tube is further divided with 2 outer walls on the left and right, an inferior wall, near the rectum, and a superior wall, toward the bladder. Now imagine that the walls of the tube described above are divided in half the long way, a right half and a left half. The left half corresponds to the clock at 1, 2, 3, 4, 5, 6 o'clock, and the right half corresponds to the 7, 8, 9, 10, 11, and 12 o'clock positions.

The Goddess Clock Stretch

To review, twelve o'clock is by the clitoris, six o'clock is by the rectum, three o'clock is to the left and nine o'clock is to the right. Using your finger, start stretching your vagina using the clock as visualization. Remember that the PFMs are divided into three layers, each layer corresponding to the knuckles of the finger and progressively deeper inside the vagina. The first PFM layer is knuckle one, the second PFM layer is knuckle two, and the third PFM layer is knuckle three.

WHAT TO DO:

1. Focus your stretching from 4 to 8 o'clock positions avoiding 12 o'clock where the bladder is located.

2. Start with PFM Layer 1, then progress to Layer 2, and then to Layer 3, only when you feel comfortable and confident.

3. Press around the clock for 30 to 60 seconds or until you feel a release in the vaginal muscles. You can go around the clock 2 to 3 times or you can stay on the same spot for three repetitions of 30 to 60 seconds.

4. For women who have just had babies or for those who have undergone surgeries, it is best to wait at least six weeks and get cleared by your childbirth caregiver before starting your clock stretching program.

5. The main thing is to decrease the pain as you press into the muscles. I always aim for at least 50 percent reduction in pain when I do the clock stretches on my patients.

6. Oils that can be used for stretching are vitamin E oil, Rose oil and any lubricant that is organic and alcohol-free.

Keeping the Queen Flexible with Internal Thumb Stretching

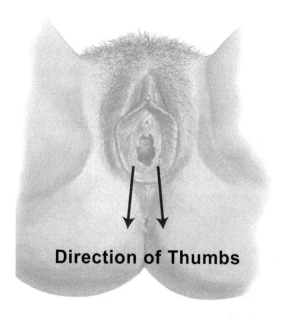

Direction of Thumbs

Direction of thumbs.
Base Image: Netter Images

This massage method works great for perineal scars, for pelvic pain sufferers with vaginismus, and also as a preparation for labor and delivery. Pregnant women can start this massage on the 34th week of pregnancy for 3 to 5 minutes. Make sure to check with your obstetrician, gynecologist or midwife before starting the perineal massage. I often teach my pregnant patients' partners to do this massage to help them prepare for labor.

WHAT TO DO:

1.   Lubricate either one thumb or both your thumbs. Insert them into the vagina up to the first knuckle, and press straight downward toward the rectum at the 6 o'clock position; hold for 3 to 5 minutes.

2. You can do this massage once a day, every other day or weekly. Some women find it incredibly erotic when their partner stretches their vagina before sex. This makes for great foreplay.

"Queen-tip" Test

So many women have pain with sex but at no other times. Others feel rawness in their vaginas and are unlikely to tolerate tampons or even panties touching their vaginas. Many go from doctor to doctor in search of answers to no avail. Sometimes there is inflammation in the vestibule and this inflammation is leading to pain and not letting us enjoy our sexual sovereignty. Inflammation in the vestibule should be checked out and can be determined by a simple Q-tip test. A nerve issue, hormonal imbalances or pelvic floor muscle dysfunction can cause inflammation in the vestibule. Most of the time this inflammation is due to a pelvic floor issue but nevertheless you should get checked out and visit a pelvic pain specialist. Many regular OB/GYNs or gynecologists are not well versed in how to treat this condition so don't go to someone who is not a vulvar pain specialist. It's frustrating and a waste of time. Many of the therapies that they might offer you are pain meds, hormones, trigger point injections, Botox injections into the vagina and/or valium suppositories. When you seek help for your Queendom you must be an educated consumer. If you are not, you fall into what I call the "Doctor Road Show," and let me tell you this is not a good place to be. It will cost you tons of money not to mention emotional distress. Save yourself the heartache and work with knowledgeable caregivers. Whatever symptoms you have or if you want to become even more aware of your body and what you can do to bring the freedom of healing to your lady parts then go to **www.pelvicpainrelief.com**/femaleFreedom. It is the preeminent online course that accompanies my Female Pelvic Alchemy book. This program provides education, guidance and practical tools along with the support of a community of like-minded women.

The Q-tip test is an essential method for determining the levels of inflammation and pain in the vestibule. As you progress on your goddess journey, you will continually perform the Q-tip test and track your results. The Q-tip test should not elicit pain. If you experience any pain with this test, consult a physician or physical therapist that specializes in pelvic pain immediately.

Where is the vestibule? The vulvar vestibule forms an oval shape around the opening of the vagina. The top is bordered by the clitoris, the bottom by the posterior fourchette, the inner sides by the hymenal remnants and the outer parts of the oval by the labia minora. Additional structures found in the vulvar vestibule include the major and minor vestibular glands, Skene's Gland and the urethra.

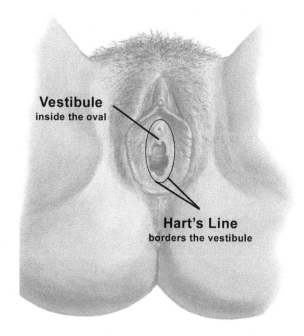

Perform the Q-tip test along Hart's Line. Source: Netter Images.

To perform this test you will need a mirror and a Q-tip with a small amount of lubricant. Locate the line that separates the labia minora from the vestibule. This is called Hart's Line. Once you locate it with your mirror, imagine the vestibule as a clock, with the clitoris at twelve o'clock, the left at three o'clock, the anus at six o'clock, and the right at nine o'clock. Using very gentle pressure, go around the clock from one o'clock to twelve o'clock. As you perform this test, rate the level of pain you experience from 0 to 10 (i.e., 0 = no pain, 5 = moderate pain, 10 = worst pain ever). If this test elicits any pain, you probably have some form of vestibulodynia. Make sure to keep track of your painful areas with your Q-tip. **And be sure to remember what I said above about being an informed vaginal consumer!**

Vaginal Scars

During your examination, you may come across old scars that you may not have noticed before. Scars and tears in the perineum can often be a source of poor pelvic strength and/or sexual pain. Vaginal scars are frequently the result of episiotomies or tearing during childbirth, or surgical procedures such as biopsies and vestibulodectomies. It is possible for the perineum to tear during childbirth or sexual activity. Check your scars for proper healing, pain and mobility. If the scar feels thick, is painful or has a discharge, have it checked by your gynecologist. If the scar is raised, painful, thick or feels tight, there are ways to reduce pain, stretch the scar, and restore motion to the tissues. In the Kegel Alchemy chapter I give additional vaginal stretches that could help you with scar tissue. Give them a try, but please do not override a pain signal. If you still have a scar that is not healing, go to your doctor and get it checked out. In the next section we will explore one of my favorite integrative therapies that helps to keep vaginas and pelvic floor muscles in perfect health.

Vaginal Steams for Vulvar/Vaginal Health

Vaginal steams were made for queens. I personally could not live without them; I find them to be relaxing and they help to balance my female energy. Vaginal steams warm up the vagina and the pelvic floor muscles and help reduce tightness and muscle spasms. Vaginal steams also help to keep us supple and flexible. Many of my patients swear by their vaginal steams and get great results with them. They experience less pelvic floor muscle tension, less pain with sitting, have easier penetration and better sex, and are able to perform their Kegels with more ease. Many tell me that the increase in circulation in their pelvis helps improve their libido. I recommend doing vaginal steams on a monthly basis. (Note: Avoid vaginal steams during your menstrual period or during pregnancy.)

I learned about vaginal steams from Dr. Rosita Arvigo, naturopathic doctor, renowned herbalist and Mayan healer. She has brought Maya Abdominal Massage to the United States and runs a great advanced certification program in Belize, which I've completed. With vaginal steams, you can mix and match the herbs and flowers you use depending on your condition. My favorite formula is rose and lavender. **Consult a local herbalist before attempting to do a steam with herbs.**

Vaginal Steam Instructions

1. Place a handful of herbs into a large pot. Add a gallon of water. Boil the water for 10 minutes and then let it steep with the herbs for 5 minutes with the lid on the pot.

2. Place water under a chair with open slats, or better yet place the bowl with the herbs into the toilet. Don't pour the steam solution into the toilet. Instead, put the whole pot into the toilet. Be

careful as it might be too hot when you sit. If it feels too hot, you can also buy a raised toilet seat to avoid burns from the steam to the vulvar area/PFMs.

3. Sit on the toilet and let the steam penetrate the PFMs via the vagina. If the steam is too hot, stand up and wait for it to cool before sitting down again.

4. Wrap yourself in a blanket, put on socks, and make sure to avoid drafts while you are doing the steam. Sit down until all the steam has evaporated, about 15 to 20 minutes.

5. While sitting on the toilet, perform deep breathing so that the pelvic muscles are evenly heated and relaxed. The steam introduces heat into the vaginal muscles, helping them to relax and reduce spasms.

6. After the vaginal steam, massage the vaginal muscles with the techniques I have shown you in this chapter and in the upcoming chapters.

7. Do your best after a steam to keep your body at a constant warm temperature for 24 hours, avoiding sudden drafts that might give you a chill.

8. Work with a local herbalist to see which flower/herb mixture might be the best for the specifics of your condition. See the following table for herbs and their uses. You will need one quart of the herbs if you are using fresh herbs and one cup if using dry herbs. The Arvigo Institute has a great formula of herbs that you can get directly from them.

Table 2.3 Herbs That Can Be Used in Your Vaginal Steams

Note: This list is for educational purposes only. You must consult your physician or herbalist before using any of these herbs in a vaginal steam. These herbs should not be taken by pregnant and lactating women unless prescribed by your caregiver. The information in this table comes from www.mountainroseherbs.com.

Calendula	Helps to reduce pain naturally. Its antibacterial, anti-inflammatory, antifungal, and immuno-stimulant properties help treat slow-healing cuts. It soothes irritated, burning skin and also helps to stimulate collagen synthesis.
Basil	Helps restore immune function deficiency caused by stress. It also has antibacterial properties and helps other herbs penetrate the skin.
Motherwort	Helps with menstrual tension by acting as a uterine tonic. This herb has antibacterial, antifungal, antispasmodic, antiviral, and antiseptic properties.
Oregano	This herb has antispasmodic, antiviral, and antiseptic properties.
Rosemary	This herb has antioxidant, antiseptic, and antispasmodic properties. Helps to stop yeast from growing and helps to remove yeast cells from the urinary tract. Stimulates menstrual flow. Avoid this herb if your flow is already heavy.
St. John's Wort	This herb helps relieve pain. Should not be used together with Monoamine Oxidase Inhibitors (MAOIs) or Protease Inhibitors (PIs). Also helps to slow down frequent urination and can treat throbbing pain of any origin.
Lavender	This flower helps to reduce tension and tightness in the pelvic floor muscles.
Lady's Mantle	This herb helps to tone the pelvic floor muscles.

Vulvar Care: Basic Vulvar Skin Hygiene

As a child I was not taught vulvar care. It surprises me to this day that many of us still don't know how to treat our vaginas with proper care. Irritation and burning of the vulva and vagina are common among women suffering from pelvic floor muscle dysfunction. There are many things you can do to minimize these feelings in your vulva. The following is a list of recommendations that have worked for my patients. Remember: these are only recommendations and you must find the ones that are appropriate for you and your condition. If you have any doubt, please show the list to your caregiver to make sure that you practice what will work best for you.

Recommendations for Better Vulvar Care

1. Although it may seem obvious, always wipe from front to back after urination and bowel movement to avoid infections.

2. Keep the vulvar area dry. Pat dry the vulva; do not vigorously rub it with towels or toilet paper. If the vulva is irritated, use a blow dryer set on cool or let it air dry.

3. Sleep in the nude at night. My patients find sleeping in the nude helps reduce their irritation. The oxygen is wonderful for the female tissues; whenever possible expose your vulva to air.

4. Avoid irritants such as perfumed soaps, bubble bath, feminine hygiene products and colored toilet paper on the vulva. If you must use soap, try something gentle and fragrance-free or try calendula soap. Also avoid getting shampoo on the vulva. There is a whole industry that is making money from us because we think our vaginas smell and need to be constantly cleaned. But there is no reason to use soaps on our vulvas. We have a natural odor that is wonderful.

5. Use unscented white and chlorine-free toilet paper, and whenever possible, use organic toilet paper.

6. Use menstrual pads and tampons that are perfume-free and 100 percent cotton. Make sure to use the appropriate tampon size for menstrual flow. During light days, use tampons with lighter absorbency, and during heavy days use super absorbency. Again whenever possible, use organic products and avoid deodorized sanitary pads and tampons. You can even use a menstrual cup if tampons and pads irritate you.

7. Avoid pushing with urination and defecation. Avoid constipation by drinking enough water for proper hydration and taking in enough fiber. Staying properly hydrated helps keep the urine diluted and makes it less likely to irritate the vulva and the bladder.

8. After urinating, rinse the vulva with cool to lukewarm water. A perineal bottle (spray bottle) works great, especially after childbirth. Alternatively, you can invest in a bidet for your home.

9. Avoid douches unless prescribed by your caregiver. Douches can upset the natural balance of organisms in the vagina.

10. Avoid chlorinated water and avoid swimming in pools. Patients have experienced terrible flare-ups after being in chlorinated pools.

11. Perform vaginal steams once a month and/or on the day after your menstrual cycle ends.

Helpful Tips for Relieving Vulvar Pain

1. Extra virgin coconut oil works great on irritated vulvar skin. Apply a small amount of the oil to the vulva as needed to protect the skin. It also works for women who experience increased friction in the vulvar area with walking.

2. Calendula cream applied to the vulvar area will help soothe irritated skin. Use on another body part first to make sure you are not allergic to it. Calendula is derived from a flower and is used to soothe skin inflammation. You can also use a calendula wash and soap, which is described later in this chapter.

3. Too many times my patients use over-the-counter anti-yeast treatments that only make the burning and irritation worse. Do not use over-the-counter creams, ointments and anti-yeast medications without consulting your caregiver first. Prescription medications like Diflucan™ can get rid of yeast infections without irritation to the vulvar-vaginal area. I also like garlic cloves. Many times when I have yeast I insert a garlic clove in my vagina and change it every 4 hours and it works like a charm. Remember that garlic is a powerful antibiotic. I use it for 3 to 5 days before I consider taking any medications. Boric acid tablets and calendula vaginal suppositories also work great for yeast.

4. To soothe vulvar burning, some women find relief by applying witch hazel pads (TUCKS Pads). These pads are also a lifesaver after giving birth.

5. Taking lukewarm to warm baths helps with vulvar itching and burning. Fill the bath tub with a few inches of lukewarm to warm water and add colloidal oatmeal such as Aveeno™ to help reduce itching. Alternatively, try adding 4 to 5 tablespoons of baking soda to the bath to soothe vulvar itching and irritation.

6. Use sitz baths to relieve burning and irritation. A sitz bath is a bath in which the hips and buttock are submerged. Usually a small basin is used and placed on top of the toilet. After childbirth, using a sitz bath with Epsom salt can help reduce pain and prevent infections. You can also steep calendula flowers and add the calendula water to your bath as well.

7. Apply a cool compress for 10 to 15 minutes to the vulva to help decrease pain and irritation. This technique is great if you have had a recent flare-up or severe vulvar pain.

8. Extra virgin coconut oil helps to rejuvenate the vulvar tissues and makes an excellent sexual lubricant. Make sure it's extra organic. You can add a small amount of water so that it penetrates the vulvar skin better.

Common Treatments for Your Queendom

The perineum is an extremely sensitive area of the vulvar region that often undergoes trauma, especially during childbirth, when women may experience perineal tearing and episiotomies. Sometimes these wounds do not heal properly or do not heal at all, and continue to open up with intercourse, defecation and exercise. For persistent perineal wounds that do not seem to heal properly, work with your doctor or caregiver to find the right combination of medicines and vitamins that will complement your perineal stretching and scar mobilizations. The following is a list of remedies that my patients have tried with positive results, but make sure to work with your doctor to be certain of the combination that is right for your specific needs.

Vitamins to Improve Skin Conditions of the Perineum

To be taken internally and under the supervision of a healthcare professional:

1. Vitamin C
2. Vitamin A
3. Vitamin D
4. Vitamin E

Alternative Massage Oils and Creams for the Perineum

1. Vitamin E oil: organic if possible.

2. Rose oil and "Down There Oil": This is a special oil that I have personally developed and I see dramatic improvements in my patients' vulvar tissue with consistent use.

3. Estriol bioidentical hormone helps with dryness due to prolonged breastfeeding and hormonal changes. It's a lifesaver for many women that I treat.

4. Calendula cream is very soothing and works well for vulvar irritation. You can also make a sitz bath out of calendula flowers to relieve pain and itching or to maintain vulvar health.

5. Extra virgin coconut oil is great as a vulvar cream and also as a sexual lubricant.

Vulvar Care and Clothing

1. Avoid wearing pantyhose. Use thigh- or knee-high hose instead. If you must wear pantyhose, cut the crotch out.

2. Double rinse any clothes that come in contact with the vulva. Wash clothes with organic detergents. Avoid fabric softeners and dryer sheets on all clothing that comes in contact with the vulvar area. Whenever possible use organic, fragrance-free detergents.

3. Remove wet clothing immediately, especially after swimming and wash the vulvar area with water as soon as possible to avoid burning and inflammation that many times comes with swimming in a chlorinated pool.

4. Avoid wearing very tight jeans, pants and clothes made from synthetic fabrics that capture sweat and increase irritation. Also avoid low-rider jeans that can put pressure on the bladder area. Instead choose a pair of jeans that are loose and baggy in the crotch area and around the waist.

5. Try wearing 100 percent cotton underwear. Many of my patients find that thongs increase vulvar irritation and can also irritate the anal area.

Managing Vulvar Pain and Bladder Discomfort after Sexual Intercourse

1. Use water-soluble lubricants for sexual intercourse. When possible, use only organic products.

2. Urinate after sex. Many women can develop bladder infections after sex. I believe that this "bladder infection" is often related to tight pelvic floor muscles, trigger points or spasms in the pelvic floor muscles. Many times during sexual intercourse if the bladder is dropped far enough into the pelvis, this feeling of bladder infection can be activated. However, this is oftentimes not a true infection. Before taking any over-the-counter medications or calling your MD, use an over-the-counter testing kit to check yourself for a bladder infection.

3. Rinse the vulva with cool water after sex.

4. Apply a cold compress to the vulva immediately after sex to reduce irritation. Apply compress for at least 15 to 20 minutes for better results. Repeat every hour as necessary.

5. Lidocaine, commonly prescribed by doctors, helps reduce pain during sex. Lidocaine can sometimes burn for 3 to 5 minutes after application. I would use this as a last resort because if there's

pain in the vulva you need to address this and not just numb the pain. Many doctors love to prescribe Lidocaine, vaginal trigger point injections and Botox, but those interventions should be used only after other treatments have been exhausted. Proper vulvar care and a good pelvic health program will go a long way in relieving if not resolving pelvic pain.

6. Focus on "outercourse" or tantric sex instead of intercourse when you are in pain. Experiment with lap dancing, oral sex, massage, mutual masturbation. Old-fashioned kissing can go a long way when you cannot have sexual intercourse. There is an obsession with penetrative sex that has to be overcome. There is so much more to sex than just a penis going into a vagina. Keep yourself open and encourage your partner to do the same.

7. If you are having intercourse, make sure you are both fully aroused and well-lubricated to reduce the actual penetration time and pain.

8. Make sure to stretch before sexual penetration to reduce pain and/ or to enhance sensation and increase the power of your orgasms. Too many times my patients contract their muscles out of fear or habit right before intercourse, which increases their pain. Keep your pelvis in neutral alignment if you are on the bottom. Do not rotate your hips back; this will make your pelvic floor muscles tighter and we want your pelvic muscles to be open and supple.

9. Experiment with different sexual positions to see which ones are the least painful and which ones bring you the most pleasure. Sometimes being on top can let you control the depth of penetration during sex. Place a couple of pillows under your buttocks so you are not engaging in full penetration. Again I cannot stress that if there's pain with sex you need to find another way to express intimacy. Pain with sex is just not worth it for many reasons.

10. You can also place your vibrator inside the vagina and gently massage the muscles with low vibration. This vibration helps to get the muscles to release and perform better during sex.

Exercise and Vulvar Care

1. Avoid exercise that puts direct pressure on the vulva, such as biking and horseback riding. If you must bike, use padded pants and a padded seat or a bike seat designed to alleviate pressure on the pelvis such as the BiSaddle™, which has two mini seats built into one. Also try to limit the length of time you spend biking in general. This includes Soul Cycle, spinning and any other type of biking that increases pelvic soreness or pain. Consider massaging your vagina after biking to ensure vaginal suppleness and better orgasms.

2. Low-impact exercises such as walking are great because they don't create a lot of friction in the vaginal area. For some, walking is not enough to really get their hearts pumping. High-impact exercises are acceptable as long as they don't increase leaking, pressure or pain. The best advice is to find cardiovascular exercises that don't increase gluteal, hip or low-back muscle spasms, and/or bladder and vaginal symptoms. Cardiovascular exercise is important on a daily basis as it helps decrease stress, elevate natural endorphin levels (natural pain killers), and keep the heart and mind healthy. However, you have to find a balance so that you don't worsen any painful symptoms.

3. Avoid exercising in synthetic materials that do not breathe, capture sweat and increase vulvar irritation. Use cotton materials. Wear loose-fitting clothes and change your underwear immediately after exercise.

4. Perform the techniques in this book on a daily basis, especially the vaginal stretching which will help reduce your pelvic pain.

5. Use a cool pack or ice pack on the vulva after exercising if pain or tension increases. Wrap the cool pack up with 1 to 3 towels so that you don't cause damage to this very gentle skin. Cool packs and ice packs can be left on for 15 to 20 minutes.

6. Avoid classes like spinning and kickboxing which can throw out your hip and sacral alignment and put excessive pressure on the perineum. Practice your reverse Kegels so you can maintain your focus on your pelvic floor as you do your exercises. If you do attend these classes, use the pelvic corrections in Chapter 6.

Castor Oil Packs

Castor oil has been used for medicinal purposes dating back to ancient Egyptian times. It is derived from the bean of the ricinus communis plant (also called palma christi because of its palm-shaped leaves and its miraculous healing properties). Introduced by Edgar Cayce, the father of modern holistic medicine, castor oil packs are the external use of castor oil and are commonly used by alternative healers for a variety of conditions and health problems. Castor oil packs promote healing of the tissues and organs underneath the skin. They help increase blood and lymphatic flow, relieve constipation and decrease congestion of abdominal organs. Additionally castor oil packs can improve the autoimmune system, relieve pain from arthritis and tendonitis, and are used to break up scar and abdominal adhesions. For pelvic-pain patients castor oil packs are commonly used to decrease pelvic congestion by improving blood circulation to the abdominal organs. Many women use them to break up adhesions after abdominal surgeries. Others use the packs to treat fibroids, ovarian cysts and to improve fertility.

WHAT TO DO:

1. Soak flannel or cotton material in castor oil so that it is thoroughly soaked and saturated but not dripping wet.

2. Place the pack over the affected body part. Cover the castor oil with plastic. Place the hot water bottle or heating pad over the pack. When using a heating pad, put it on the medium to high setting. Do not fall asleep with the heating pad on. Make sure to use a heating pad with an automatic shut-off button.

3. Leave it on for 45 to 60 minutes. Rest while the pack is in place. This is a great time to meditate and/or practice your reverse Kegels.

4. For non-acute conditions it is generally recommended to use a castor oil pack 3 times per week, every other day. On the fourth week, rest and do not apply a castor oil pack. Consult with your healthcare provider for your specific treatment regimen.

5. After removing the pack, cleanse your skin with a diluted solution of water and baking soda.

6. Store the pack in a covered container in the refrigerator. Each pack may be reused up to 25 to 30 times and can last for 6 months.

WHAT TO WATCH OUT FOR:

1. Castor oil should not be taken internally, as it is a harsh laxative.

2. Castor oil packs should not be applied to broken skin.

3. Castor oil should not be used on C-section or abdominal scars before 6 weeks. Consult your doctor before applying a castor oil pack to your scars.

4.   Castor oil packs should not be used during pregnancy, breastfeeding, or during menstrual flow.

With the integrative therapies we have explored in this chapter, you have been exposed to the benefits of acupressure therapy and have taken the time to examine yourself and learn about the importance of vulvar care. That's great progress! Now let's move forward to the next chapter where we look at how and why you may be experiencing problems in your queendom...

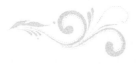

You have come this far, but I have more to teach you.

Taking Care of Your Lady Business Naturally

...to go deeper ONLINE, visit
http://www.FemalePelvicAlchemy.com/chapter2

Many of the techniques discussed in this book have been
videotaped and are part of my online program.
In the training video designed to accompany this chapter,
I share with you something special that will help you
to go deeper into understanding your "Queendom."
This video is not to be missed.

CHAPTER 3

The Wayward Goddess

We all know that if things are going well in the Queendom, then all is well throughout the land. But what if things aren't going well? What if the Queendom has issues? If you consider your personal Queendom, you will agree that if you have pain and discomfort in the pelvic area, your whole body feels the impact.

So what may be the cause of your Queendom issues? More specifically: what has made your goddess behave in a wayward manner? This is a loaded question, one that has brought many queens to their knees.

Chances are you may have felt something not quite right in your lady parts. Maybe you sought help from your MD only to be told: "this is normal" or "have a glass of wine and relax." (I have heard the most unhelpful comments from members of the medical profession.)

Before we can bring peace to the queendom, we must understand that the vagina is a complex ecosystem with muscles, nerves, arteries, fascia, and bacteria all living in incredible balance. So of course when things go wrong "down there" repercussions are seen throughout the entire female system. A wayward goddess needs special attention to bring her back home to herself. One of the biggest problems that I currently see in women's health is a lack of knowledge about the pelvic floor muscles and what happens when these muscles are not in optimal health. Remember that the pelvic floor muscles live within the vagina, and this is where they can be assessed and examined. Because these muscles support our pelvic organs, control our continence, are involved in sexual function, pelvic bone stability and bowel function, they can create havoc—confusing most clinicians—when they are behaving waywardly. The pelvic floor muscles are also intimately connected to our pelvic nerves, blood supply and energetic systems. I will cover this in more detail later in the book, but for now what I really want you to understand is that although you may be experiencing problems, all is not lost. Sometimes the solutions to your lady parts issues are simple and do not require medication, surgeries or exploratory exams. Many times working within the vagina with massages and exercises can bring profound relief and symptom reduction.

To determine whether your goddess is wayward, first review Table 3.1 and take note of whether or not you have experienced any of the symptoms that are described.

Table 3.1 Typical Symptoms of a Wayward Goddess

Origins Of Symptoms	Symptoms As Reported By My Patients
Emotional (usually in combination with other symptoms)	- Catastrophic thinking - Isolation - Strained relationships with partners - Depression - Sadness - Guilt - Sleep disturbances - Suicidal tendencies/thoughts - Emotionally unavailable
Muscular	- Pain in the gluteal or back muscles, knees, or abdominal area - Generalized soreness in PFM muscles - PFM spasms - PFM trigger points - Constant or sharp-like pains in muscles associated or near the vagina - Pelvic floor muscle weakness
Rectal	- Bleeding with defecation - Constipation - Pain with defecation - Redness around the anus - Burning-like pain - Itching - Pushing to get feces out - Feelings of pelvic pressure - Pain in the rectum after orgasms - Pain or irritation with thong underwear

Dermal (Skin)	- Allergies to metals, perfumes - Sensitive skin - Irritation with certain toilet papers, tampons or sanitary napkins - Itching - Sensitivity to soaps - Painful scars - Feelings of vaginal swelling - Burning pain in the labia - Constant ache throughout the vulva - Raw feeling in the vaginal tissues
Vaginal	- Painful intercourse - Vaginal itching, burning, rawness - Constant awareness of vaginal area with certain clothing - Pain with touching/wiping - Pain at opening or deep inside - Clitoral pain - Labial pain - Cuts in the vagina - Skin patches of varying colors - Pelvic pressure – feels like something is falling out of the vagina
Urinary	- Painful urination - Urgency and frequency of urination - Suprapubic pain - Hesitancy in getting urine out - Slow urine stream - Feelings of incomplete emptying - Habit of pushing urine out - Vaginal stinging with urination - Urethral pain - Feelings of pelvic pressure - Leaking with coughing, sneezing or laughing

If you have any of the symptoms I described, you might be suffering from one of the many medical conditions that affect the pelvic floor muscles. Of course it is my recommendation that you seek medical attention when needed from a specialist who is well versed in female conditions and the pelvic floor muscles. Make sure to follow up with a second and even third opinion. If all the exams are negative and you have no systemic or localized diseases, then you are probably suffering from pelvic floor muscle dysfunction.

Medical Conditions Affecting the Pelvic Floor Muscles

What are the most common conditions? Most cases fall under the umbrella of vulvodynia, vestibulodynia, dyspareunia, vaginismus, interstitial cystitis, pudendal nerve neuralgia, lichen schlerosis, endometriosis/fibroids, and scar pain. Let's take a moment to examine each of these conditions. Most of my patients have some combination of conditions that are contributing to their wayward goddess. As you take a look at each condition, you may very well discover that your symptoms point toward multiple contributing factors. Don't worry. First and foremost, we need to separate and identify each factor that is causing your pain so that you can devise the best approach to attacking and ultimately defeating the pain that is controlling your life right now. Many times you will need manual massage therapy to the vagina. I cover these massages in Chapter 7. Other times you may need a Kegel/reverse Kegel program. Understanding the different types of medical conditions that can affect the pelvic floor muscles is key. Once you have figured out that these muscles are involved, this book will provide you with some excellent techniques and tools. My ground-breaking book, *Ending Female Pain,* is another excellent resource for any woman whose goddess has gone astray.

Vulvodynia

Vulvodynia is an umbrella term used to describe pelvic pain. There are actually several variations among which it is important to draw a distinction. Many of my patients have difficulty pinpointing their vulvar pain. They say it hurts "everywhere down there," which is called generalized vulvodynia. For others, the pain is at specific spots in their vulvas such as in their vestibules, which is called localized vulvodynia or sometimes called vestibulodynia. For some, their pain is worse during and right before their periods, or pain comes on all of a sudden, which is called unprovoked vulvodynia. Pain is sometimes also felt with direct contact to the vagina such as when wiping or with sexual intercourse. This is called provoked vulvodynia. Many also report they cannot have any penetration because the penis cannot get in the vagina (vaginismus).

The causes for vulvodynia are largely unknown and are thought to be multi-faceted. There is no evidence that vulvodynia is caused directly by sexually transmitted diseases or infections. Recent research has put a lot of emphasis on the nerves that innervate the pelvic and vaginal area, indicating that vulvodynia is a result of a neuropathic condition where the nerves are not functioning properly. Whatever the root cause, many gynecologists, urologists and caregivers agree that the pelvic floor muscles are deeply affected, and many times normalizing their function can bring great relief to pelvic pain sufferers.

Childbirth

Childbirth is a major culprit of sexual pain and pelvic floor muscle dysfunction in women. The pelvic floor muscles are stretched to their limits during delivery and the pelvic nerves also undergo traction and stretching, often compromising their function. While these are all natural occurrences during birth, once coupled with perineal tears, episiotomies, Cesareans, and assisted deliveries using vacuums and forceps, the birth trauma can be quickly compounded.

In obstetrics and gynecology pelvic trauma during birth is classified into degrees of tears. A first-degree tear is a tear through vaginal mucosa and perineal skin only; a second degree tear is a tear that extends into the pelvic floor muscles; a third degree tear involves a tear that extends into the external sphincter; and a fourth degree tear is a laceration affecting the anal sphincter and anal rectal mucosa. No matter what the level of the tear I believe that women should be routinely referred to a pelvic floor specialist after birth, and most definitely uro-gynecological rehabilitation should be prescribed to all women after pelvic surgeries. In many other countries, such as France, pelvic rehab is routinely prescribed to new moms, but in the US this is not the common practice.

New moms come to me with varying complaints including pain with sitting while breastfeeding, pain with sexual intercourse, urinary leaking, fecal incontinence, perineal scar pain or Cesarean pain. To facilitate recovery after childbirth, I emphasize pre-natal pelvic education to solidify strategies for success.

Expectant mothers need to know that perineal massage started religiously at 34 weeks of pregnancy is a great preparation for labor and helps prepare the PFMs for the upcoming stretching during labor. It is also very important for pregnant women to choose a healthcare provider who will not routinely perform episiotomies unless absolutely necessary. Pregnant women also need to be empowered with information and made aware that certain positions are less likely to cause perineal tearing and obstetrical trauma. For example, the lithotomy position (on your back) has been correlated with the highest rate of pelvic tearing. I also find that this position compromises the pubic bone and many women suffer from Symphysis Pubic Dysfunction when they labor on their backs or when their legs are pulled apart too aggressively. Surprisingly the side-lying birth position is the safest for the pelvic floor muscles. You should have a say as to what position you will use for giving birth. You are the queen, and everyone must remember that. Make sure to let your pregnant friends know that they should choose wisely when picking a caregiver to help them to deliver their baby. I urge you to get a doula. A doula can help and guide you through your pregnancy, delivery and post-partum period. Also, my online *Female Pelvic Alchemy* program is great for any woman who wants to heal from pelvic pain and pelvic floor muscle dysfunction. With my guidance, you will see that there are things you can do to help yourself.

Vestibulodynia

Vestibulodynia is a localized, provoked form of vulvodynia, in which particular areas of the vestibule show certain characteristics. The vestibule is the oval-shaped area around the opening of the vagina. This condition, sometimes also called vulvar vestibulitis, is one of the most common sexual pains I treat. Vestibulodynia is characterized by three criteria that were first proposed by researcher E.G.Friedrich, Jr. in 1987, in the *Journal of Reproductive Medicine, 32:110-114.* The 3 main characteristics as described by Friedrich are:

1. Pain when the vestibule is palpated with a cotton swab. This is called the "Q-tip test" and is described in greater detail in this book in the section on vaginal self-examination.

2. Erythema or redness throughout the vestibule that can sometimes extend to the labia majora and inner thighs.

3. Severe pain with vaginal penetration of the penis, speculum, tampon, finger, or dilator.

Be aware that some healthcare practitioners don't use these criteria, but you should keep these characteristics in mind in case this comes up during your gynecological exams.

The pain felt in the vestibule is thought to be caused by a proliferation of intraepithelial nerve endings found in the vestibular mucosa. Research also shows that these nerve endings contain a compound called calcium gene-related peptide. This compound is found in C-fiber nerves which are present in the vestibule. The research indicates that women with vestibulodynia have 10 times more C-fiber pain nerves in the vestibules than normal women. It is thought that this increase in C-fiber nerve endings is one of the major culprits contributing to the excruciating pain felt by women suffering from this condition.

Another possible culprit is the hyperactivity of mast cells in the vestibule. These cells play a part in the inflammatory process and also produce, among other compounds, nerve growth factor which is thought to help turn normal nerves that process pain signals into neuropathic nerves that produce pain signals no matter what the external stimulus may be.

Sometimes vestibulodynia is due to an imbalance in female hormones and can even be caused by the birth control pill. Getting women off the pill is one of the first things I try if they suffer from vestibulodynia. Many times vestibulodynia is caused by very tight pelvic floor muscles. Many of my patients sometimes use vaginal valiums, hormonal creams or nerve-suppressing medications to help the vestibule to calm down. These medications will not work unless the pelvic floor muscles are normalized and their long-held tension, spasms and/or trigger points are addressed. Other women get Botox in their pelvic floor muscles to get them to soften again.

Vaginismus

Vaginismus occurs when the muscles of the pelvic floor go into involuntary contraction, creating spasms that close the vaginal opening. Usually the first sign of vaginismus is an inability to insert a tampon.

Patients with vaginismus find it difficult, if not impossible, to have sex because of severe spasms in the outer layer of the vagina. Pain in the hips, lower back, and gluteal muscles is reported as well, which makes daily activities challenging. These patients have sexual desire but the contracted muscles do not allow the penis to enter into the vagina without pain. Vaginismus is best treated with manual stretching of the pelvic floor muscles and with medical dilators. With proper self-care, the affected muscles release their spasms and trigger points and become softer and more supple, making sexual penetration possible. Many queens have difficulty consummating their marriage and this adds a tremendous amount of stress and duress to the married couple. I have seen many women come in crying after their lovers have left because of their pelvic pain. Any man who doesn't understand that the goddess goes wayward sometimes is not worth it.

Fibromyalgia

Fibromyalgia syndrome affects the muscles, tendons, ligaments, and soft tissues of the body. Patients generally complain of pain throughout the entire body, including the vulvar and pelvic/hip region. Additional symptoms include extreme fatigue, sleep disturbances, and burning sensations throughout the body. Fibromyalgia sufferers have multiple trigger points and tender spots all over their bodies that when pressed elicit pain. To diagnose fibromyalgia, a good physician relies on a detailed medical history, and checks for pain and tenderness in 11 out of 18 specified trigger point areas along with locating painful areas in the body that have persisted for more than three months. For more detailed information about fibromyalgia visit a great online resource called *www.FMaware.org.*

Interstitial Cystitis

Interstitial cystitis, or IC, is a medical condition that produces pain in the bladder and urethra. IC is also known as painful bladder syndrome, and patients with IC often report symptoms of pain in the vulva, pain with intercourse, and pain in the lower back and hips. Other common complaints include urinary urgency – a feeling of an urgent need to urinate, or urinary frequency. Sometimes, the frequency can be extreme. I have had patients who go to the bathroom every 5 to10 minutes. Another common symptom is pain when the bladder is full, and patients often report that the pain subsides after urination. I recommend my IC patients keep a food diary, as there are many bladder irritants that can lead to painful flare-ups and contribute to excruciating pain if consumed. Here is a list of foods to avoid if you have been diagnosed with IC:

1. Fruit juices such as orange, cranberry, tomato, or lemon juice are bladder irritants.

2. Caffeine stimulates bladder nerves, causing pain, inflammation, and irritation to the bladder. Increased bladder nerve stimulation will also produce an increase in urinary frequency.

3. Regular or green teas because of the tannic acid found in them.

4. Regular and diet sodas because of citric acid, artificial flavoring, preservatives, and carbonation.

5. Artificial sweeteners are thought to be bladder irritants.

6. Chocolate and cocoa products may irritate the bladder lining.

7. Wine and alcohol are potential bladder irritants.

All patients with painful bladder syndrome respond well to pelvic floor therapy, and it's a critical component of the healing journey that should not be overlooked. For more information on IC, visit Jill Osborne's amazing web portal at *www.IC-Network.com*. She has done a great job of providing all of the latest information.

Dyspareunia

Dyspareunia refers to painful intercourse. This pain can occur before, during, or after sexual activity. There are many causes of dyspareunia including atrophic vaginitis, vulvar vestibulitis, lichen schlerosis, endometriosis, scar adhesions, and psychological trauma such as sexual abuse. Dyspareunia responds well to vaginal massages and pelvic floor therapy. Many of the exercises in this book well help also.

Endometriosis

I treat many women who experience sexual pain as a result of endometriosis. The uterus is lined with a specific tissue called endometrial epithelium stroma. When this tissue grows outside of the uterus it is called endometriosis. This condition can cause a lot of pain and many other problems in a woman's body. Endometrial tissue can be found anywhere in the pelvis, such as the ovaries, uterus, fallopian tubes, intestines, bladder and colon. Most women with endometriosis usually experience pelvic pains during their menstrual cycles, but many also have excruciating pain that is not related to their periods. Endometriosis can cause not only sexual pain but also infertility, as the tissue growths can affect fallopian tubes, ovaries and the proper functioning of the uterus.

If adhesions and scar tissue related to endometriosis build up, it can lead to a condition called frozen pelvis. If you think you are suffering from endometriosis you must make sure you are comfortable with your caregivers. Visceral manipulations, cranial scar therapy and pelvic floor therapy are natural ways to deal with pain associated with endometriosis. My online *Female Pelvic Alchemy* program is great for any woman who wants to heal from pelvic pain and pelvic floor muscle dysfunction.

Adhesions/Scar Pain

Post-surgical scar adhesions occur in women after most pelvic and abdominal surgeries. An adhesion is a fibrous band of scar tissue that forms between internal organs and tissues, joining them together abnormally. Adhesions form after surgery as part of the normal healing process and help to limit the spread of infection. Sometimes though, adhesions cause tissues to grow together that normally would not be connected. Millions of people worldwide suffer from painful adhesions after surgery, and data has suggested over 50 percent of women will develop scar adhesions following gynecologic and non-gynecological surgeries *(Obmanagement.com, June 2003, Vol. 15, No. 6)*. In my experience, the longer a woman waits to seek therapy for her scars, the denser and tougher the scar adhesions become. More importantly, scar adhesions may be associated with pelvic pain and sexual pain, abnormalities of bowel function, and infertility.

I have seen many women develop overall pelvic pain because of adhesions after surgical procedures such as C-sections, myomectomy, hysterectomy, laparoscopic procedures, episiotomy, vestibulectomy, hymenectomy, perineal tearing, and even vulvar biopsies.

Sexually Transmitted Diseases (STDs)

Sexually transmitted diseases (STDs) also negatively affect the PFMs leading to dysfunction and/or pain. PFMs should never be massaged during active infections. Learn to recognize the following STDs and seek medical help right away if you think you may have one.

1. Herpes presents as tingling, itching at first and then painful sores.

2. Chlamydia Trachomatis is a bacteria that can form sores or ulcers. Most common STD.

3. Gonorrhea can present as a foul-smelling discharge.

4. Syphilis can present as sores in the vagina and anywhere in the perineum.

5. Human Papilloma Virus is characterized by a discharge or open sores.

6. Chancroid produces sores in the genitals with swollen genital lymph nodes.

Infections

There are some infections that affect the pelvic area. These include:

1. Bacterial Vaginosis (Gardnerella Vaginalis) is a bacterial infection associated with a foul, fishy odor.

2. Trichomonas vaginalis is a parasite that is typically asymptomatic. When women notice symptoms it is because they cause urethritis, an itching, burning and discharge from the urethra.

Lichens Planus

Lichens Planus is a common inflammatory disease involving the skin and mucous membranes that affects adults and can involve any portion of the body, but it has a tendency to surface in the wrists, ankles, and oral and genital tissues. It is characterized by small, flat-topped many-sided bumps (polygonal) that can grow together into rough, scaly reddish purplish plaque. It can cause extreme vaginal itching. There is no known cure and treatment is focused on controlling the itching. The PFMs can respond by becoming tight and inflexible.

Lichens Sclerosis

Lichens Sclerosis is a skin condition that mostly affects the genital and perianal areas. It is characterized by small white, shiny, smooth spots on the skin that grow into bigger plaques that become thin and wrinkled. The lesions can be reddish or purple in the acute state and then turn white when the condition is chronic. I have seen chronic cases where there are very large patches of white all over the vaginal area.

The skin can easily tear leading to vaginal scarring and causing the vaginal opening to get small and constricted. The PFMs also contract and become inflexible in response to the itching and pain. Many women complain of extreme itching that can lead to blisters and bleeding. Many believe it is an autoimmune issue and the treatment can involve steroid cream or ointment.

Pudendal Nerve Neuralgia

Pudendal Nerve Neuralgia (PNN) is a shooting, stabbing and knife-like pain in the distribution of the pudendal nerve. The pudendal nerve has a very unique anatomy and journey within the pelvic rim that makes it vulnerable to becoming entrapped, compressed or irritated by fascia, muscles, scar tissue, ligaments and surgeries of the pelvis. One of the leading causes of PNN is myofascial dysfunction. A woman's pudendal nerve can become injured during gynecological surgeries that include repairs for rectocele, cystocele and hysterectomies. Childbirth can also result in injuries of the pudendal nerve. Additionally the pudendal nerve can be injured during bike riding, falls, accidents, coccyx injuries, etc. Pain can be localized to the clitoris, labia, vagina, vulva, rectum, sit bones or perineum. Symptoms can be unilateral or bilateral but usually there's a more affected side. Pudendal Nerve Neuralgia pain can get worse with sitting and many women find relief with pudendal nerve block. Pain does not wake them up at night and they usually have no sensory deficits. Some patients can have increased sensitivity (hyperalgesia), allodynia (increased pain to non-painful stimuli), or parathesia (tingling or numbness). Physical therapists successfully treat the pain, spasms, tight muscles, trigger points, connective tissue restrictions, scars and joint dysfunction that contribute to symptoms of PNN. If you are suffering from PNN, you will benefit greatly from pelvic floor therapy.

After reading this chapter, it should be clear that there are many reasons why you may be experiencing a wayward goddess. Because pelvic pain can be complicated and involve multiple systems, addressing it requires a multidisciplinary integrative approach. Luckily for you, that is exactly what I have to offer you. Continue reading and I will show you…

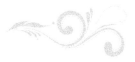

You have come this far, but I have more to teach you.

The Wayward Goddess

…to go deeper ONLINE, visit
http://www.FemalePelvicAlchemy.com/chapter3

In this special training video, I go even deeper and guide you
through techniques and tools that help you to understand why
your goddess went wayward. Once you have this knowledge,
you will feel like you are coming home, back to yourself
in a way that makes sense for you and your life.

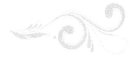

CHAPTER 4

The Harmonious Bladder

So many women have bladder issues that affect their sex lives and self-esteem. And guess what? We don't have to live that way! The bladder, in my opinion, is easily trainable. You don't have to suffer from embarrassment, and you don't have to worry that you will leak during sex. There are things you can do to get the bladder back into harmony. Even if you don't have bladder issues the information I provide for you here will increase your goddess IQ. The better informed you are the more confident you will be with your body. I am all about empowering women and this chapter takes the mystery out of the leaky temperamental bladder and helps to put an end to all the misconceptions about getting our bladders into alignment with our lives. In this chapter I will discuss how to manage your bladder by sharing "real deal" bladder information that will consist of massage and helpful tips to put your bladder back on track.

The bladder has many connections to different parts of the body, including the anterior wall of the pelvic floor muscles. These connections occur via fascia, nerve and muscle. Your bladder should hold about 300 to 500 ml of urine, which correlates to about 10 to 16 ounces. When the bladder is full it sends a message to your brain signaling that it is ready to be emptied. When you void you should empty to a very low volume and there should be no feelings of incomplete emptying. Experiencing these symptoms is an indicator that your bladder needs training and that there is also a dysfunction within the Pelvic Floor Muscles (PFMs). Additionally there should never be pain, urge, post-dribble leaking or a need to push the urine out with voiding. If these dysfunctional voiding patterns are not corrected, they will create havoc and misery in your life.

Remember that the bladder and the PFMs talk to each other, so if the bladder decides to behave badly, the PFMs will also start to misbehave. For the bladder to empty completely the PFMs need to be able to relax and let go. If the PFMs have trigger points, spasms and/or poor coordination, then there is a higher risk for bladder dysfunction. Conversely, when the PFMs relax, the bladder contracts, but if the bladder starts to contract or spasm inappropriately or at the wrong times, that can lead to urge, leaking with urge and an increase in frequency. Before you know it you have become a slave to your bladder and you are looking for a bathroom everywhere you go. Urge leakage can happen at any time, but many patients report that it occurs around a certain activity. For instance some complain of "key in the door" syndrome: they start to get the urge and leak as they open the doors to their homes. With the trade secrets highlighted in this chapter and throughout this book I am certain you will resolve many of your bladder issues.

Hands-On Techniques for Better Bladder Health

If I had a dollar for every time that I found bladder urge and pain stemming from the muscles of the legs, butt, or abdominal area, I would have a lot of money. In this section I will cover the body parts that you need to investigate for bladder symptoms. I will also give you several amazing exercises and tools that will help you to resolve your bladder dysfunction. The areas of interest here are the inner thigh muscles, the suprapubic abdominal muscles and the sacrum. Many times these areas are loaded with trigger points that are referring to the bladder; you have to resolve these trigger points to get the bladder back under control.

Suprapubic External Bladder Trigger Points

Although the points that I will be discussing here are not true acupressure points, when you work on the suprapubic points you start to get your bladder urge, incontinence and/or pain under control. Incorporating these points into your goddess self-care program is a true game-changer. Many of my patients complain about pain right above the pubic bone. They also complain of burning and that low-rider jeans make them want to pee. There's a reason for this. The bladder lives underneath this bone. It makes sense that if there is a dysfunction in the bladder that the top of the pubic bone and the lower abdominal area will be painful and filled with trigger points. The following technique brings about amazing results and can help reduce bladder urgency. Many times trigger points in this area refer pain to the bladder. This is one of my go-to techniques for women suffering from bladder conditions.

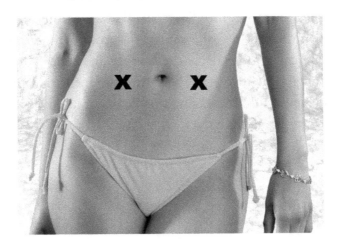

WHAT TO DO:

1. Start your investigation by pressing along the top of the pubic bone and your lower abdominal muscle area. Take note of where the pain is and what symptoms you feel when you press into these areas.

2. Make yourself a simple map. Note pain level from 0 to 10 (0 = no pain, 10 = worst pain) and symptoms produced.

3. Hold the trigger point for 90 seconds, making sure to release the trigger point slowly. Repeat as many times as necessary until the pain level is reduced by 50 percent or you feel relief from the symptoms.

4. CAUTION: Do not press into an area that has a pulse. If you feel a pulse, move to a different area.

Bladder Up-Glide Massage

Not only will bladder massage help to normalize bladder behavior, it will also affect the Conception Vessel Ren points discussed in Chapter 2. So this massage is a win-win for the bladder and will help you bring back your sexy. There are three ligaments that arise from the umbilicus like a tripod and attach to the superior aspect of the bladder. These ligaments are called collectively the urachus ligaments. They have to function well and help with the upward movement that the bladder undergoes when it fills. Massaging this ligamentous area is important for bladder health and function.

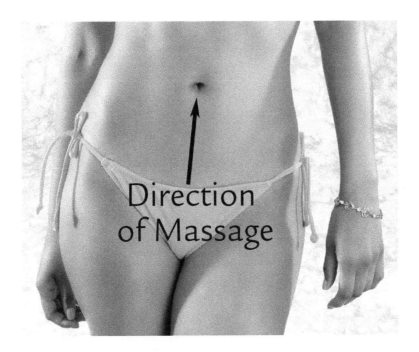

WHAT TO DO:

1. Place your fingertips on the top of your pubic bone and massage upward toward the belly button.

2. Maintain firm but gentle pressure as you massage upward.

3. Repeat for 30 strokes. If you discover a trigger point along the way make sure to take care of it by pressing into the trigger point for 60 to 90 seconds.

Inner Thigh Trigger Point Release

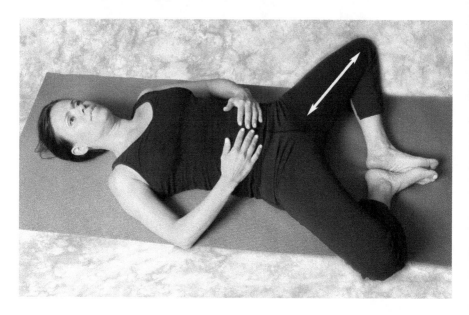

The inner thighs are the gateway to the Queendom. That is one of the reasons why we can become so fixated on them, toning them with exercise and obsessing about thigh gaps. The inner thighs are an erogenous zone for many women and massaging them helps to improve vaginal tone and circulation. The inner thighs connect to the vagina via the pelvic floor muscles. So when I want to have a deep effect on my patient's sexual function I will explore these muscles with vigor. And normalize them. Spasms and pain in the inner thigh muscles have a direct connection to the bladder and pelvic floor muscles and require special attention. The inner thigh muscles can develop spasms, trigger points and adhesions in them as a response to what is happening internally in the bladder or in the vagina. These tissue abnormalities can lead to bladder urgency and pain. The trigger points in the inner thigh can refer to the bladder and they can also refer to the vagina. A trigger point will feel like a hard, small ball and will produce pain when touched. In terms of the bladder a trigger point in this area may also give you urge.

WHAT TO DO:

1. Examine your inner thigh muscles by sweeping your hands over them. You are searching for trigger points, spasms or areas that give your bladder symptoms.

2. Once you find them, press into the trigger points for 90 seconds until the pain has diminished or gone away. You may have to do several cycles of 90 seconds to accomplish this.

3. Complete normalization of the inner thigh is necessary because this muscle is a major culprit in creating bladder symptoms such as urgency and bladder pain.

Psoas Release

The Queen has met her king. In my opinion, the psoas is the king of all muscles. This muscle has a direct connection to our sexual energy chi and can help improve not only our sexual health but also bladder function. This is one of my go-to muscles for almost anything related to the Queendom. If there's pelvic congestion, low back pain, bladder issues, fertility issues, low libido and/or sexual dysfunction, I make sure this muscle gets its just desserts.

The psoas is a very deep muscle located on either side of the lower abdomen. The psoas muscles attach from the lower spine to the hip bones, and help flex the hips. In women suffering from pelvic pain, sexual dysfunction, poor bladder health and weak orgasms, the psoas muscles are frequently very painful, in spasm, and irritated. The kidneys have an intimate connection to this muscle. Keeping the psoas muscle pain free, supple and flexible is critical for improving our goddess power.

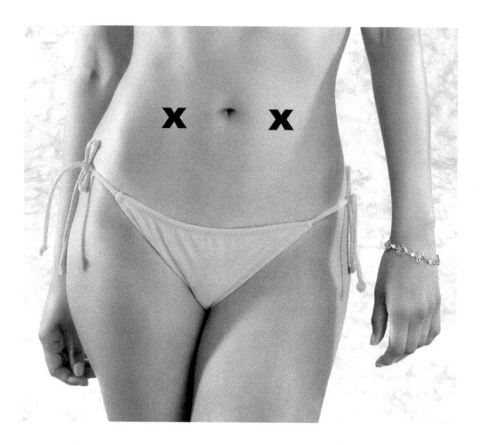

WHAT TO DO:

1. Lie on your back with your legs straight out.

2. Go about two to three inches to the right side of your belly button. Place your fingertips into the area, slowly allowing them to sink into your abdomen and being careful to avoid any feelings of an artery pulse.

3. Lift your right leg straight up and you will feel the psoas pop into your hand. It may take a little practice to get this but keep trying. Once you know where the psoas muscle is, place your fingertips in that spot and slowly press downward into the psoas for 60 to

90 seconds. If you feel any tingling, numbness, or tremendous **increase** in pain, get off the area and try to relocate the psoas muscle. Switch sides and do the left psoas muscle release.

4. CAUTION: Do not press into an area that has a pulse. If you feel a pulse, move to a different area and locate the muscle at another place.

The Successful Bladder: What Every Goddess Should Know

Urge control and suppression techniques are important because they not only buy you time to get to the toilet dry but they also help to retrain the bladder back to health. This will take time so don't become discouraged if at first you can't beat your urge; with time and practice you will.

Controlling Your Urges

1. Cross your legs and put pressure on the urethra when the urge hits.

2. Perform a quick Kegel contraction. Start with 10 and continue until the urge has subsided. Be careful not to go into PFM spasms.

3. Apply pressure on the perineum or clitoris.

4. Slow down your pace and move slowly. Do not rush or run to the bathroom.

5. Begin deep diaphragmatic breathing and continue breathing this way until the urge subsides.

6. Distract your mind from the urge. Occupy yourself with another activity or think of something else.

7. Tighten your gluteal muscles and curl your toes under. This helps to shut down the nerves that innervate the bladder.

8. Keep your body as warm as possible. Cold stimulates the bladder.

9. Don't slouch; keep your body upright and arch your back slightly to reduce pressure on the bladder.

10. Loosen your pants or shirt tops to reduce pressure on the bladder.

11. Keep in mind that your bladder responds to what you eat and drink.

What You Eat Impacts Your Bladder

Diet makes a difference in your bladder symptoms. Urine is composed of water, toxins, and substances that your body is trying to eliminate. When you have an injured bladder, urine can reach deeper in the bladder walls stimulating nerves that trigger inflammation and irritation. By adjusting diet, no matter how hard it may be, you will be able to calm the bladder down so it can heal.

Table 4.1 Four Food Types That Cause Irritation

Foods high in acid (ex: orange juice, cranberry juice)	Consuming highly acidic food and/or drink is comparable to pouring salt on a wound.
Foods that stimulate nerves (ex: caffeine in coffees and teas)	If frequency of urination is an issue, food and drink that triggers nerves in the bladder will worsen the issue.
Foods high in histamines (ex: chocolate)	These foods can trigger an allergy-like reaction.
Foods high in sodium or potassium	A lesser cause of triggering pain; however, some patients experience a reaction.

Table 4.2 The Top Seven Foods to Avoid and Why

Coffee	The caffeine in coffee triggers nerves and irritates the bladder.
Regular and Green Tea	The caffeine and the flavoring tannic acids in regular tea irritate the bladder. Green tea is highly acidic.
Soda and Diet Soda	Citric acid, flavoring, preservatives, artificial flavoring, and acidity in all sodas irritate the bladder. The caffeine also triggers nerves.
Fruit Juice	The acidity of fruit juice irritates the bladder. Pear and apple juices may be acceptable.
Multivitamins	The body cannot use the massive amount of vitamins found in supplements and they are excreted out of the body through urine. Vitamin C (Ascorbic Acid) and Vitamin B6 are notorious for irritating sensitive bladders.
Artificial Sugar	For an already injured bladder, artificial sugars create profound irritation.
Chocolate	Chocolate is notorious for triggering allergies and also causing pain in an already irritated bladder. Carob, a chocolate substitute, is usually an acceptable and delicious alternative.

Table 4.3 The Top Seven Foods to Promote Bladder Wellness

Meats	Be wary of spicy, preserved meats such as pepperoni and salami. Avoid meat sauces.
Veggies	Eat your veggies! However, steer clear of acidic tomato products. In some cases, asparagus cause irritation.

Dairy	Go for milk and eggs. Eat cheese with caution sticking with mild, fresh varieties like mozzarella, cottage cheese, or soft Monterey jack. Avoid highly spiced cheeses like pepper jack.
Breads	Stick with fresh, preservative-free, simple breads such as wheat, oat, white, and rice. Steer clear of rye and sourdough breads.
Fruits	Start with fruits low in acid such as pears and blueberries. A mild apple, mango, papaya, and melon can be introduced slowly.
Desserts	Treat yourself, on occasion, to vanilla ice cream with caramel sauce. If you need your chocolate fix, explore your dessert options using carob, a chocolate substitute.
Herbal Tea	Sip on peppermint or chamomile herb teas. The next step would be introducing carob roasted teas then moving forward to herbal coffees.

A Final Piece of Diet Advice

Eliminate manufactured foods and junk food. Buy organic as these foods are less contaminated with pesticides and chemicals which could irritate the bladder. No matter how hard it is to stick with this new way of living you have to try. It's not a forever kind of thing. Once you have brought your bladder back into harmony you can then introduce these foods back into your life. This is a temporary commitment until your bladder gets back to normal. Focus on your healing. Making changes is hard no matter who we are but we have to give it our all. We can't half commit. Being a true goddess is about finding balance and doing what is necessary to get back to the Queendom.

Goddesses Track Their Bladders

A picture paints a thousand words and your bladder diary will enlighten you and help you to figure out where you need to focus. Sometimes when we are deeply suffering or when our bladders are just a big old mess, we forget to check in with ourselves and take a good look at our habits and behaviors. A bladder diary is key if you want to retrain and control your bladder and finally stop the leaking, pain or constant peeing. To get a great idea of what's going on with your bladder I recommend that you keep track of your bladder for one day during the week and for one day during the weekend. (We behave differently when we are away from the stresses of our jobs and our week day routines.) Your diary will paint a picture for you and you will get the clarity and the information that you need to retrain your bladder and finally learn how to stop your bladder from controlling your life. The bladder is an easy organ to control, but you have to be diligent and relentless. Start right away. You may have to keep this diary for several weeks because it is just as important to track your progress over time so you can reward yourself when you hit certain milestones.

Keeping a Record of Bladder Function

A bladder log can give you an excellent picture of your bladder functions, habits and patterns. At first, the log is used as an evaluation tool. Later, it will be used to measure your progress on bladder retraining or leakage episodes. **Please complete a bladder log every day for 2 days (i.e. one work day and one weekend day).** Normal bladder fitness is 6 to 8 voids per day, at least an 8 Mississippi urine stream with a 3 to 4 hour interval. There should be no leaking and only a normal urge to void. I know this bladder data may be shocking for some of you but this is what you are moving toward. You can do this. Your log will be more accurate if you fill it out as you go through the day. It can be very difficult to remember at the end of the day exactly what happened in the morning.

INSTRUCTIONS

Column 1 - Time of Day
The log begins with midnight and covers a 24-hour period. Afternoon times are in bold. Select the hour block that corresponds with the time of day you are recording information.

Column 2 - Type & Amount of Fluid (EXCLUDING WATER) & Food Intake

- Record the type and amount of **fluid (EXCLUDING WATER)** you drank in ounces.
- Record the type and amount of **food** you ate.
- Record when you woke up for the day and the hour you went to sleep.

Column 3 – Amount of WATER Intake

- Record the amount of water you drank in ounces.
- The recommended amount of water for a 24-hour period is 6 to 10 cups or ½ your body weight in ounces.
- If you find you are drinking less than the recommended amount, your bladder may be more irritated which can increase urgency, frequency, and leaking!

Column 4 - Amount Voided (Urinated)

- When voiding, count the number of seconds you void by using the counting convention "One Mississippi, Two Mississippi, etc…"

- Record this number in the appropriate row corresponding to the correct time.
- Record a bowel movement with a BM at the appropriate time.
- You should be voiding > 8 Mississippi's per void. Anything less will disrupt the bladder and its associated reflexes.

Column 5 – Urgency Level/Leakage

- Record the level of urgency just prior to voiding.
  - Was the urge HIGH (H)? – "Oh my God, I almost didn't make it!"
  - Was the urge MEDIUM (M)? – "I really had to go but didn't necessarily need to rush."
  - Was the urge LOW (L)? – "I casually made my way to the bathroom."
- Did you leak urine? Record (Y) for Yes, and (N) for No.
- If yes, what activity were you doing? Coughing? Sneezing? Running? Post-urination dribble? Or was it just that the urge was so strong that you leaked?

Daily Voiding Log Sample

Time Of Day	Food/Liquid (Excluding Water): Type Of Food & Drink	Water Intake (Ounces)	Amount Urinated (In "Mississippi's)	Urge Present? (L / M / H) Leaking? (Y / N) Activity With Leaking?
Midnight				
1:00 am				
2:00 am				
3:00 am				
4:00 am				
5:00 am				
6:00 am	Woke up at 6:45 am		8	M
7:00 am	Coffee, bagel			
8:00 am				M
9:00 am	Apple		10	
10:00 am				
11:00 am			6	H – Y leaked before I got to toilet
NOON	Tuna sandwich, milk, pear			
1:00 pm				
2:00 pm			8	M
3:00 pm	Tea, cookies			
4:00 pm				
5:00 pm				
6:00 pm	Chicken, corn pudding, salad, apple juice		10	L
7:00 pm				
8:00 pm				
9:00 pm				
10:00 pm	To bed at 10:30		12	M
11:00 pm				

Number of Pads and/or Panty Liners Used: _____

How would you describe your urinary stream? (Put an X in all that apply)
- ☐ Hesitant – Difficulty Starting
- ☐ Slow / Weak
- ☐ Angled to One Side – Circle One: (R) or (L)
- ☐ Stop / Start During Void
- ☐ Painful – Before (Y / N) ; During (Y / N) ; After (Y / N)

Daily Voiding Log

Time Of Day	Food/Liquid (Excluding Water): Type Of Food & Drink	Water Intake (Ounces)	Amount Urinated (In "Mississippi's)	Urge Present? (L / M / H) Leaking? (Y / N) Activity With Leaking?
Midnight				
1:00 Am				
2:00 Am				
3:00 Am				
4:00 Am				
5:00 Am				
6:00 Am				
7:00 Am				
8:00 Am				
9:00 Am				
10:00 Am				
11:00 Am				
Noon				
1:00 Pm				
2:00 Pm				
3:00 Pm				
4:00 Pm				
5:00 Pm				
6:00 Pm				
7:00 Pm				
8:00 Pm				
9:00 Pm				
10:00 Pm				
11:00 Pm				

Number of Pads and/or Panty Liners Used: _____

How would you describe your urinary stream? (Put an X in all that apply)
- ☐ Hesitant – Difficulty Starting
- ☐ Slow / Weak
- ☐ Angled to One Side – Circle One: (R) or (L)
- ☐ Stop / Start During Void
- ☐ Painful – Before (Y / N) ; During (Y / N) ; After (Y / N)

This chapter has shown you that normalizing your voiding interval and eliminating foods that irritate the bladder are as important as doing the correct Kegels and restoring your core strength. I have given you the tools to achieve holistic bladder health; make the most of them and you will be rewarded with long-term positive results. Now let's take a look at how to build a strong foundation for pelvic health.....

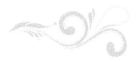

You have come this far, but I have more to teach you.

The Harmonious Bladder

…to go deeper ONLINE, visit
http://www.FemalePelvicAlchemy.com/chapter4

When the bladder is unhappy, it can bring a queen to her knees. Whether you seek to overcome your bladder madness or are just looking to increase your goddess IQ, be sure to check out the training video that corresponds to this chapter.

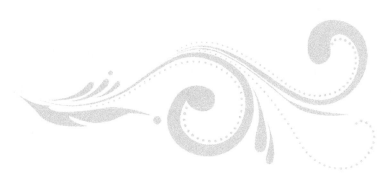

CHAPTER 5

Reclaim Your Womanly Foundation

*I*t is the simple things in life that matter the most, and many times it is the simple adjustments that we make in our lives that have the most impact. Many women experience pelvic pressure, incontinence, organ prolapse, and sexual dysfunction. *If you are one of these women, you don't have to suffer:* all you need is some guidance. There are things you can do to protect yourself and to keep your symptoms in check. These behavioral changes will also improve your goddess IQ and confidence. I am going to share with you my trade secrets, information that most doctors, osteopaths, physical therapists and other healthcare professionals learn from experience or through their studies while in school.

Over the last ten years I have treated thousands of women, and when I share with them my trade secret list they are astonished. Why? Because my list succeeds where other methods have failed. My trade secret list has been created with the woman in mind, and the suggestions and modifications in this list are a game-changer. When you implement my trade secrets into your everyday living you will notice that you can carry your body better, you will feel more in control, and most importantly, you will be able to enjoy life.

The Trade Secret List

At my healing center and my online pelvic healing school, one of the first educational materials we give our patients is a comprehensive trade secret list, which encompasses the basic rules and precautions all women need to know to stay healthy, strong, and prevent injury. As you read through my trade secret list note what changes *you* need to make. Not only do I share with you what to avoid but I set you up for success and triumph by telling you what to do and how to do it. You will experience freedom from pelvic symptoms and feel like your old self again after you implement my suggested changes.

Table 5.1 The Trade Secret List— Tried-and-True Strategies

What To Avoid	Trade Secrets To Use
Jackknife out of bed	Log roll out of bed
"Valsalva" maneuver breath holding	Breathe naturally focusing on exhale
Push with urination or defecation	Use the proper potty posture
Just in Case (JIC) Urination	Avoid all JIC voids and keep a bladder diary
Bend forward from the waist when lifting heavy objects	Use proper lifting mechanics
Poor sitting posture	Use correct sitting posture
Poor standing posture	Use correct standing posture
Impact exercises	Walk and listen to your body
Don't let it all hang out	Protecting the Goddess: Use the "Pelvic Brace" (a simultaneous transverse abdominal contraction and Low Level Kegel)

Avoid Jackknifing Out of Bed

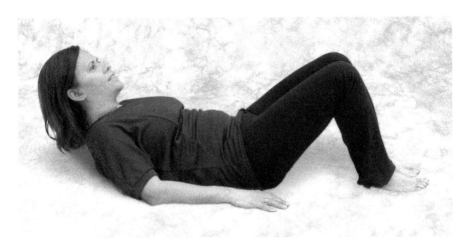

Description: Notice the tension in the abdominal, neck and upper back muscles. Jackknifing also strains the abdominals and causes them to open up like a zipper at the linea alba.

Jackknifing is the act of sitting up straight out of bed as if you were doing an abdominal crunch exercise. Jackknifing puts your abdominal muscles under a lot of stress and strain and can lead to a condition called diastasis recti. The rectus abdominis muscles are joined at the middle by a connective tissue sheath called the linea alba. When you jackknife you put a lot of stress on the linea alba, and like a zipper, it can open at the seam creating a gap.

For more information on diastasis recti abdominis (DRA) and for an in-depth analysis of how to test and correct for it, see the core chapter. If you have ever seen a bulge that pops out in the middle of your belly, especially during positional changes, this is a DRA bulge. DRA is bad news and needs to be contained. One of the easiest modifications you can do is to avoid poor body movements such as jackknifing. Also avoid forward bending from the waist, which is a form of standing jackknifing.

Trade Secret to Use: Log Rolling

To avoid making a DRA bigger and putting excessive stress on your abdominal area, simply log roll out of bed. To log roll, turn completely to the side first, and then use your arms to help you sit up along the edge of the bed. Log rolling is less stressful for the abdominal muscles and will help prevent the diastasis from getting any bigger and wider. **Additional tip:** If you are suffering from pubic bone or groin pain, squeeze a pillow between your knees while you roll to the side. This helps to stabilize the pelvis and hip bones and can significantly reduce pain during these difficult transitional movements.

Avoid Holding Your Breath

A "Valsalva" maneuver or holding your breath places increased stress and strain on the abdomen, pelvic organs, and pelvic floor muscles. The Valsalva maneuver is defined as a forced expiration of air through a closed glottis. Holding your breath, when lifting objects or having a bowel movement, can cause your pelvic organs to descend placing increased pressure through the pelvic floor muscles. When your organs descend they can prolapse and lead to pelvic floor muscle dysfunction, incontinence or pelvic pressure. Holding the breath can even make your DRA wider and contribute to abdominal weakness, herniated disc and back pain.

Trade Secret to Use: Focus on the Exhale, Grunt and Moan

Focus on the exhale with all your activities to reduce stress and strain on your pelvic organs, abdominals and lumbar pelvic region. It is helpful sometimes to count out loud when you are performing your exercises and other daily activities.

Don't Push with Urination or Defecation

Do you ever feel as if you need to push or strain when you have a bowel movement or urinate? This destructive force can be detrimental to your pelvic floor muscles. When you push or strain to go to the bathroom, the abdominal organs actually descend downward resulting in a large amount of stress through the muscles of the pelvic floor. The cumulative effect of pushing and straining when going to the bathroom can make you susceptible to pelvic organ prolapse, weakened pelvic floor muscles, incontinence, and pelvic pain. It is extremely important to limit the amount of stress through the pelvic floor and limit pushing as much as possible.

Trade Secret to Use: Potty Posture

Potty posture is the ultimate position for better bowel and bladder function. Before I started using potty posture I just never felt right about my bathroom habits. The potty posture puts your body, pelvic floor muscles, bladder, colon and internal organs in the best position for emptying. Most importantly proper potty posture helps to relax your pelvic floor muscles facilitating the best possible bowel and bladder function. My patients swear by it and so will you.

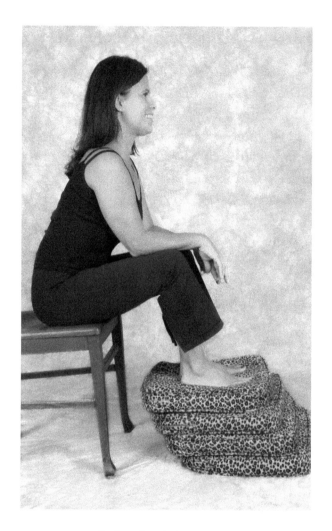

Proper potty posture includes the following steps:

1. Sit with your knees above hips, legs wide apart and feet plantar flexed, which means on your toes. For women less than five feet tall, use a footstool or book if necessary. Taller women may not need to elevate feet to maintain the position.

2. Lean forward and place your elbows on your thighs. Keep the arch in your back and avoid slumping or rounding the lower back.

3. Gently bulge out your abdominals while simultaneously widening your waist as if to "brace" yourself from a blow to the abdomen.

4. Once you can bulge and brace simultaneously this can be used as a toilet technique, as it will help relax the pelvic floor muscles and facilitate defecation.

5. Avoid straining. Do not hold your breath. As mentioned earlier, play with sounds such as "*Ohhh*," "*Ahhh*," and "*Shhh*," which will help further relax your pelvic floor muscles. Correcting your potty posture takes time, but with practice you will master it.

Constipation is another unspoken destructive force for women. Constipation, straining and pushing with defecation or urination creates havoc for your "down there" muscles and you must avoid it at all costs. To manage constipation make sure you are getting the right amount of fiber, drinking plenty of water, and always using the correct potty posture. Don't forget to discuss with your doctor, midwife, or healthcare provider how to manage your constipation so that you don't put excessive stress on your pelvic floor muscles and internal organs.

Avoid Just in Case (JIC) Urination

We are all guilty when it comes to "Just in Case" (JIC) urination. I myself wasn't even aware that I was doing it until I started to take note of my bladder habits by tracking them with a voiding log. JIC can adversely affect the way your bladder functions causing you to have to use the bathroom frequently. JIC can also lead to nocturia: waking up at night to use the bathroom. When your bladder fills to its volume, a signal gets sent to your brain which then stimulates your body to urinate by getting an urge. Many women go to the bathroom before they get a proper urge leading to "shrinkage" of the bladder. Hence the expression: "I suffer from a small bladder." Women do *not* have small bladders. Going to the bathroom before the bladder fills and before you get the proper signal to urinate can lead to urge, urge incontinence and frequent trips to the bathroom. Normal bladder function is six to eight voids per day every three to four hours with no leaking. A normal void lasts for approximately eight to ten seconds. If your voids are shorter than that duration, you are experiencing some dysfunction and you need to correct for it.

Trade Secret to Use: Use Time Voiding, Bladder Diary and Waiting for Proper Urge

A picture paints a thousand words. To get the real scoop and to see the truth you must keep a voiding log and take note of what is going on with your bladder. Review Chapter 4 and keep these tips in mind:

1. Avoid bladder irritants such as carbonated drinks and caffeine.

2. Stay hydrated; do not limit your water which can lead to bladder dysfunction including urge, urge incontinence and stress incontinence.

3. Fill out a bladder diary (see Chapter 4) to normalize your bladder function and regulate your voiding intervals.

4. Listen to a proper urge and avoid all JIC urination.

5. Don't push to get the urine out. Don't do it. You will do more harm than good.

Avoid Bending Forward from the Waist

My husband blew out his back when my baby was three weeks old. I kept after him: "Please don't bend from the waist" and "Please bend from your knees to put the baby in her crib." He did none of that, and one day when he was bending over to put our daughter into her crib, he couldn't stand up again. Low and behold, he herniated his disc and that was a disaster. He was in pain for several weeks, so not only did I have to care for my young daughter but now I had a severely injured husband.

Making new habits and breaking faulty patterns is difficult. So difficult that many of us find it an agonizing process when it comes to change.

One of the best ways to protect your back from injury is to use proper mechanics and to bend from the knees and not from your waist.

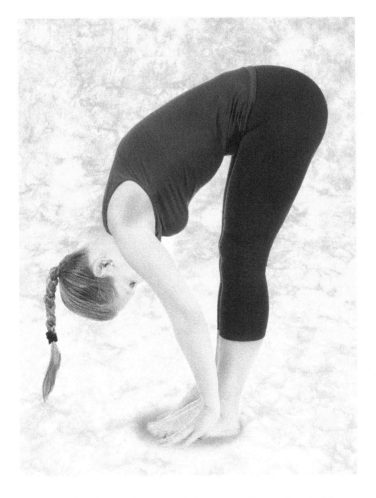

Description: Bending forward incorrectly increases the mechanical forces on the spine and increases the likelihood of injury.

Body mechanics—the way someone moves when carrying and lifting objects—can have a huge impact on the joints and muscles in the neck, back, hips, and legs. Improper mechanics over time can lead to conditions such as cervical or lumbar disc herniation, sacroiliac joint pain and instability, hip bursitis, muscle spasms, and generalized low back and hip pain.

Bending forward from the waist with a rounded back places increased stress on the discs in the spine. Intervertebral discs lie between each lumbar vertebra, or bone, in the back. The discs act as cushions that support the back and absorb impact forces. They've been compared to jelly donuts: There is an outer ring, which is made up of tough connective tissue and helps to contain the nucleus. This nucleus, or the jelly in the donut, is a water-based substance which acts as the cushion in the system and helps to absorb and distribute forces. When you bend forward and round your back, it is like *"smushing"* one side of a donut against the plate. If you do this once in a while and without too much force, the donut may bounce back to its original form and be just fine. However, if you do this over and over, or smash the donut against the plate, the jelly squirts out the other end and your donut is ruined. This is similar to what can happen to our lumbar discs if we repeatedly bend forward from the waist or attempt to lift a very heavy object with improper body mechanics. A disc affected in this way is described as herniated; herniated discs can cause severe pain in the back, and sometimes numbness or tingling, into the legs (often referred to as sciatica).

Trade Secret to Use: Proper Body Mechanics

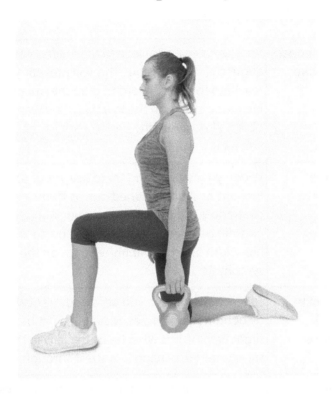

Description: Improper body mechanics can place undue stress on the back and hips and increase risk for intervertebral disc herniation. Do not bend forward from the waist. Instead bend from the knees and use proper biomechanics.

Proper lifting mechanics can feel awkward at first and may be challenging to your body. Follow these simple guidelines to help minimize the stress on your back and hips. The sooner you begin to practice proper lifting mechanics, the better your body will be prepared to lift and carry without putting yourself at risk for back or hip injury.

Table 5.2 How to Lift Properly and How to Use Proper Body Mechanics

Bring the Load/ Object Close	Bring your body as close to the load/object you are about to lift as possible. This will prevent you from reaching too far forward to grab the object, placing increased stress on the low back. You want the object almost directly underneath your body before you lift it.
Wide Base of Support	Widen your stance and try to keep your toes pointed forward or slightly turned out, as if you are about to straddle the object. For women with pubic bone or groin pain, your stance should be no wider than hip-width apart to minimize stress on the pubic symphysis.
Squat Down and Bend Your Knees	To reach the object, you will need to squat down by bending your knees. Maintain a flat back with a slight arch. This is what helps the jelly in the donut stay centered, placing less stress through the discs.
Keep the Load Close	When you grasp the object, bring the load close in to your body and stand up with your back remaining straight up and down. Avoid over-reaching and putting undue stress on your spine.
Take Steps: Do Not Rotate	Do not rotate, or twist, your trunk to place the object on a different surface. Instead, take small steps with your legs to reposition your body. Set the object down using these same principles.

Avoid Heavy Lifting

We never advise heavy lifting. Lifting heavy weights—even several bags of groceries—puts a lot of downward pressure on the pelvic floor muscles and organs. Many women develop organ prolapse because they are carrying heavy weights or their older children.

Trade Secret to Use: Don't Lift Anything Weighing Over Ten Pounds

Our rule is simple: don't lift anything weighing over ten pounds. Listen to your body. If you are unable to maintain proper body mechanics, feel pain with lifting, or notice you have to hold your breath when you lift, you are most likely lifting an object that is too heavy and you should lighten the load.

Avoid Poor Sitting Posture

How many times have you been told to sit up straight or stop slouching? In today's society, more and more people have desk jobs requiring them to sit for prolonged periods. Slouching, or bad posture, can be a destructive force especially for women. Sitting postures in general result in the largest amount of pressure through the lumbar discs, as compared to lying down and standing. Slouching or slumping in your chair further increases the amount of pressure in the discs in the low back, which can exacerbate low back pain and sciatica and cause the upper back and neck muscles to become overstretched. Slouching also increases abdominal and pelvic pressure putting you at a higher risk for prolapse. Therefore, it is particularly important to improve your sitting posture to minimize stress through the vulnerable joints in your body and avoid postural-related aches.

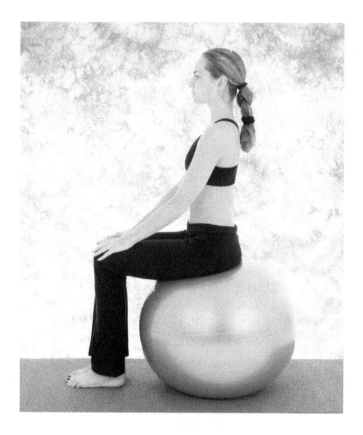

Description: This woman is in excellent sitting posture. Notice how the ears are aligned with the shoulders and the shoulders are aligned with the hips. The knees are aligned with hips creating a right angle and feet are flat on the floor. Her spine is also in neutral alignment. This is optimal sitting posture.

Table 5.3 Recommended Trade Secrets for Proper Sitting Posture and for the Work Environment

Maintain a Neutral Spine	The spine naturally should have a slight arch when sitting. However, not enough arch, or an excessive arch, can place undue stress on the ligaments, discs, and joints in the spine. Neutral spine can be achieved by rocking your pelvis back and forth as if sticking your bottom out and then tucking your tailbone under. Do this several times, and then find the midpoint between the two extremes to achieve a neutral spine. Neutral spine is our recommended position for the lower back.

Use a Lumbar Roll	Roll a towel into a cylinder and place it in the small of your back to help you maintain neutral spine and take some of the load off the back while sitting. It may take some trial and error to find the right size and texture towel to fit your spine properly. A lumbar roll can also be purchased online or in an office supply store.
Proper Hip, Knee, and Foot Positioning	The hips, knees, and feet should all be at a 90 degree, or right, angle with the feet resting flat on the floor. If your feet do not reach the floor, consider resting your feet on a step stool in order to maintain contact with the floor and place less stress through the hips and knees.
No Leg Crossing Allowed: Keep Your Feet Flat on the Floor or on a Stool	Crossing your legs can cause you to lose neutral spine and create asymmetry through the pelvis. Plant your feet flat on the floor with equal weight through both sit bones to maintain neutral spine.
Keyboard or Computer Position	The position of your keyboard should allow you to have relaxed shoulders, elbows at 90 degrees tucked close to your waist, and most importantly, a neutral wrist position. Keep your wrists flat when typing or using the mouse.
Preventing Neck and Upper Back Pain	Forward head posture and rounded shoulders are two major causes of upper back, shoulder, and neck pain. Keep your neck centered over your shoulders and chin tucked in to avoid overstretching the muscles in the back of your neck and placing increased stress through the discs. For proper shoulder position, envision your shoulder blades going down and back, as if you are going to put them into the back pockets of your jeans or pants.
Do Not Sit for Long Periods of Time	Do not sit for longer than thirty minutes at a time. Stand up, do a chest stretch, or take a walk to the water fountain as an opportunity to take pressure off the back and reset your muscles.

Avoid Poor Standing Posture: Tucked Back and Sway Back

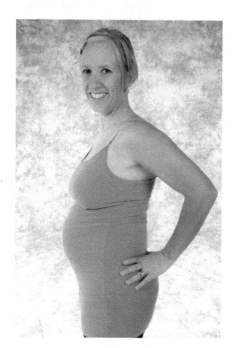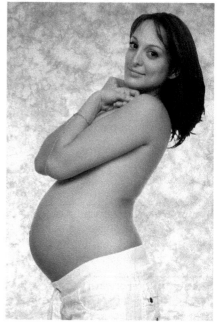

Description: The woman on the left is in a tucked-in position and the woman on the right is in a swayback posture.

There are two major postures that most women assume: "swayback" or "tucked tush." The swayback posture occurs when a woman assumes an excessive arch in the low back to maintain her balance. The tucked tush posture, on the other hand, occurs when a woman essentially squeezes the butt muscles to bring the center of gravity over the base of support in order to prevent falls. Both of these postures add stress to the lumbar spine, sacroiliac joint, hip muscles and ligaments, and pelvic floor muscles. The PFMs start to adapt to these postures and become dysfunctional, tight, short and inflexible.

Trade Secret to Use: Proper Standing Posture

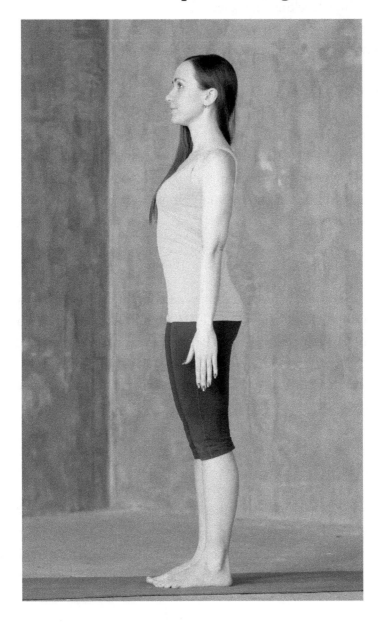

Description: This is ideal standing posture.
Notice the bend in the knees and the neck and hip alignment.

Our big trade secret for standing posture is: don't lock your knees. Why? Locking the knees throws you into a swayback posture and increases stress on your joints. Bring awareness to how you are standing and correct yourself every time you lock your knees. Keep your knees slightly bent. Another trade secret is to keep your chest lifted and your shoulders pulled back. Imagine that you are wearing a beautiful necklace and you want to show it off to everyone. Keep your head aligned with your neck; avoid forward head posture and keep your chin tucked in. The lower back should be in neutral spine position. It may seem easier to stand in poor posture, but at the end of the day your body will not be happy and pain will set in. Do yourself a favor and stand up straight.

Avoid Impact Exercises

Impact exercise, such as running and jumping, can sometimes be harmful to the body when the PFMs are not functioning optimally. If something just doesn't feel right, or if you are experiencing pain, leaking or pelvic pressure with impact exercises, you should not continue to do these activities until your PFMs are stronger and can withstand the forces produced by impact exercises.

Trade Secret to Use: Walking and Listening to Your Body's Signals

Women who have sciatica, incontinence, sacroiliac joint instability, diastasis recti abdominis, or pelvic pressure/pain should proceed cautiously with impact exercises. Women who learn that their usual body-sculpt, boot camp, Pilates, yoga, spinning, or aerobics classes may be causing and/or exacerbating their pelvic symptoms are sometimes disheartened. However, there are many alternative exercises that will help keep you active, healthy, and symptom free. A moderate-intensity walking and exercise program can help improve muscle tone, strength, and endurance, promote healthy bowel movements, increase circulation, and improve mood, energy, and sleep. Other low-impact alternatives include swimming, recumbent biking, and light weight training.

If something just doesn't feel right, listen to your body talk and discontinue the activity you are doing. Not all exercise benefits everyone, and we encourage you to become your own healer and discover what works best for your body. This principle cannot be stressed enough and is extremely important when developing your own exercise regimen. Listen to your body and don't override what it is trying to tell you.

Avoid Letting It All Hang Out

For many women with pelvic floor muscle dysfunction the abdominal muscles become stretched and weakened. Many women have no idea how to utilize their deep core muscle (transverse abdominal TrA) as a remedy for their pelvic symptoms. Many women over-activate their abdominals by over-tightening their bellies. Everyone wants those side abdominal definition lines that are considered sexy. When you try too hard to get your abdominals to kick in, you use the rectus abdominis external oblique muscles rather than the deep core muscles. Instead of letting it all hang out (or over-squeezing your core), use our trade secret and see your body shift into a more powerful position and experience less leaking, pressure and urinary urgency with your everyday living.

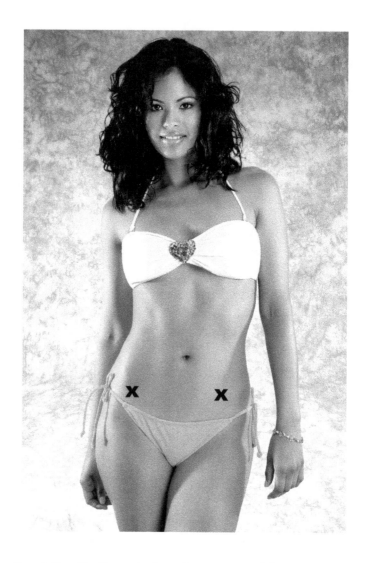

Description: The X's mark where the transverse abdominal muscles can be felt when properly activated.

Trade Secret to Use: Protecting the Goddess: Pelvic Brace (Combination of a TrA Hold plus Kegel Contraction)

The pelvic brace is your secret weapon when you are suffering from bladder, bowel and organ prolapse, "mommy tummy" or poor pelvic stability. A pelvic brace is a combination of a TrA contraction and a low-level Kegel contraction. This amazing combo exercise can help decrease back pain, stabilize the sacroiliac joint, minimize DRA, and prevent pelvic floor muscle dysfunction including pelvic organ prolapse and incontinence. All women should learn to use this pelvic brace to minimize strain through the abdomen and pelvic floor. For example, when log rolling out of bed, do a pelvic brace before you roll. Or, before you lift an object or move from sitting to standing, do a pelvic brace. This pelvic brace will help prepare the body for movements which place increased strain on the low back and pelvis, and keep your body protected. By performing the pelvic brace you can prevent injury during difficult movements throughout the day. The pelvic brace is the foundation of my core program and you must master it without overdoing it. It is an art form. (See the core chapter for more information.) I see too many women performing abdominal exercises incorrectly. Most women do not know about the pelvic brace and actually bear down and push their organs out during abdominal exercises. Many women also hold their breath when they do core exercises: couple no pelvic brace with poor breathing and you have a recipe for pelvic disaster.

Follow these steps to learn how to do a pelvic brace:

1. As you exhale, do a Kegel, or squeeze your pelvic floor muscles as if you are trying to stop the flow of urine. This ensures you will not push down on the pelvic floor muscles, and instead will initiate a lifting motion from the pelvic floor up to the TrA.

2. Draw your belly closer and more firmly toward the spine. As you pull in your abdominals try to imagine that you are trying to squeeze into an old pair of jeans that don't fit. Your belly should actually lift upward toward your nose if you perform the exercise correctly.

3. Avoid over-contracting the superficial abdominals, like the external obliques or rectus abdominis. Try to think of the TrA contraction as 20 percent of your maximal effort; it is very subtle and precise:

   - Do not hold your breath. Exhale as you perform the contraction.

   - Once you establish the above movement, hold for five seconds and repeat ten times. Do one to three sets per day to master this skill.

The goddess trade secrets I have shared with you in this chapter make it possible for you to stop your destructive forces and will help you to build a strong womanly foundation. All you have to do is increase your awareness of body positioning, posture and body mechanics. Make a conscious effort to incorporate changes and modifications into how you move your body every day and you will find that pelvic discomfort/pain will start to melt away. You will carry your body with more confidence and, as a result, you will simply start to feel better. In the next chapter, I will keep the momentum going by focusing on pelvic alignment and Kegels. Read on...

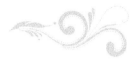

You have come this far, but I have more to teach you.

Reclaim Your Womanly Foundation

…to go deeper ONLINE, visit
http://www.FemalePelvicAlchemy.com/chapter5

Sometimes we are our own worst enemies.
This may not be intentional;
we just may not know any better. In this beautiful training
video I take you deep into what I call "Body Presence."
Check it out and you will understand that gaining control
is simple and within your reach.

CHAPTER 6

Untwist the House of Your Pelvic Muscles

*M*any of my patients come to me in search of answers they are not getting from their MDs. They tell me: "I feel like something is out of place; my bones just don't feel right; I can't be in certain sexual positions." Healthcare providers often dismiss complaints like these as an unavoidable part of being a woman. Women who suffer from prolapse, leaking, pelvic pressure, sexual dysfunction, menstrual cramps, and infertility often have alignment issues that are deeply affecting the function of their pelvis, organs and their pelvic floor muscles (PFMs). The bony pelvis is the house of the PFMs so if the bones are not in optimal alignment then the function, strength and endurance of the PFMs will also be off. It is important to note that your organs are also housed in these muscles so they will also be out of place if your bones aren't straight. Many times I will correct a patient's alignment and not only will she be less symptomatic but she also produces a better Kegel. The trade secrets I share here—secrets that are usually reserved for physical therapists, osteopaths and other rehabilitation experts—will arm you with pelvic corrections guaranteed to help you perform the best Kegel and to feel less pelvic symptoms. These pelvic corrections also help to alleviate pelvic girdle, low back or sacroiliac joint pain.

You absolutely can take steps to control your pelvic symptoms; better yet, you may be able to prevent or greatly reduce leaking, prolapse or pelvic pressure by using the tools in *Female Pelvic Alchemy*. In this chapter, I will teach you safe and effective ways for correcting your own alignment. When your pelvis is in alignment we feel connected and our goddess power increases. When your bones are in optimal alignment you will experience fewer pelvic symptoms, function better and even have better sex. Your muscles will get stronger faster because they are in an ideal position to contract and relax. You will learn how to evaluate your alignment by using simple bony landmarks. (You will first need to learn all the bony landmarks covered in this chapter to be successful with your own adjustments.) We'll begin with a review of the anatomy and function of the pelvic girdle bones.

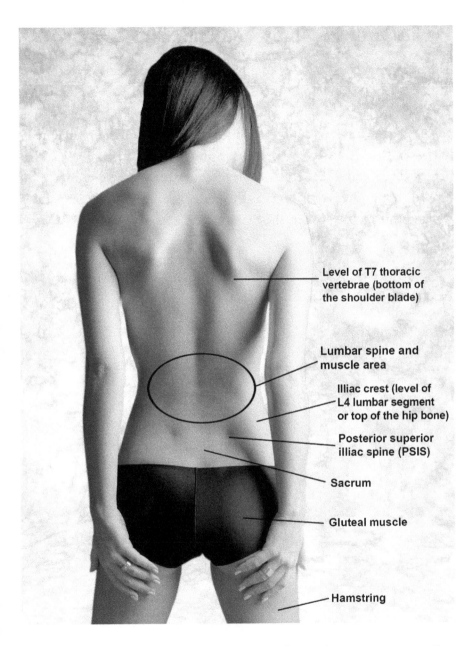

Level of T7 thoracic
vertebrae (bottom of
the shoulder blade)

Lumbar spine and
muscle area

Illiac crest (level of
L4 lumbar segment
or top of the hip bone)

Posterior superior
illiac spine (PSIS)

Sacrum

Gluteal muscle

Hamstring

Description: Surface anatomy is important to understand so you can more easily find the bony landmarks. Please take note of the different areas and keep them in mind as you read this very important chapter on how to correct your own alignment.

Pelvic Girdle Anatomy and Function

The human pelvis, which is often referred to as the pelvic girdle, is a three-part bony ring composed of one sacrum and two innominates. The sacrum is a triangular-shaped bone that forms the back of the pelvis. It is actually a continuation of the spine; however, instead of having individual vertebrae that move and flex, the sacrum is made up of five fused vertebrae. This fusion of the vertebrae results in a solid piece of bone. The sacrum acts as the keystone of the pelvic ring and is wedged tightly in between the two innominates.

Bones of the Pelvis: Anterior View of Sacrum and Innominate

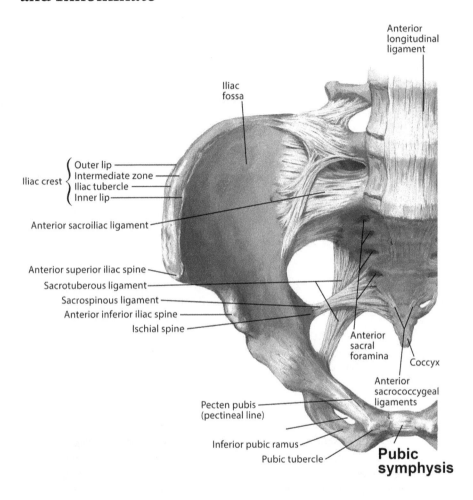

Diagram Description: This is an anterior view of the pelvic girdle. Notice the triangular-shaped sacrum. The larger bone is called the innominate and consists of three bones fused together. There is a right and left innominate bone. These bones can frequently get out of alignment in active women and women who have pelvic floor dysfunction. Source: Netter Images.

Bones of the Pelvis: Posterior View of Sacrum and Innominate

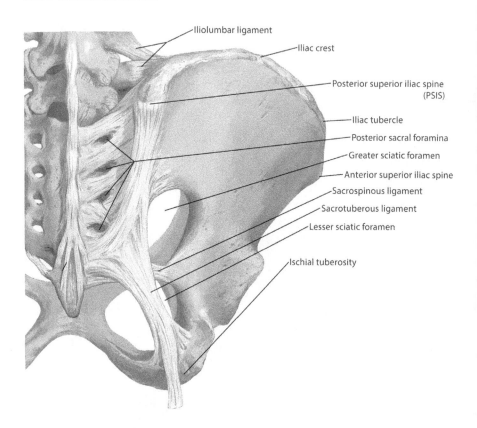

Iliolumbar ligament

Iliac crest

Posterior superior iliac spine (PSIS)

Iliac tubercle

Posterior sacral foramina

Greater sciatic foramen

Anterior superior iliac spine

Sacrospinous ligament

Sacrotuberous ligament

Lesser sciatic foramen

Ischial tuberosity

Diagram Description: This is a posterior view of the pelvic girdle. Notice the ligaments that surround and connect the sacrum and innominate. The connection between these two bones creates the sacroiliac joint. There is a left and right sacroiliac joint. It is common for women to experience pain in this joint and for this joint to get out of alignment. Source: Netter Images.

The innominates form the sides of the pelvis and are made up of three different bones that are fused (permanently joined) together: the ilium, the ischium and the pubis. The right and left innominates meet the sacrum to form the right and left sacroiliac joints (SI). The tight-fitting SI joints are designed primarily for stability and help transfer weight between the spine, legs and the ground. The strength of the entire pelvic ring is highly dependent on the stability of the SI joints.

In addition to stability, the SI joint plays a secondary role in allowing slight motion within the pelvic ring. As we walk, each side of the pelvis rotates out of sync with the opposite side of the pelvis. This opposite rotation of the innominate bones produces a torque, or torsion, within the pelvic ring. Without some flexibility of the SI joint, the pelvic ring would be too rigid to allow for walking. The faster we walk, the greater the torsions within our pelvis and the harder SI joints work to keep us moving without pain. Dysfunction at the SI joints causes pain with moving in bed, transferring from sitting to standing, walking and stair climbing.

In the front of the pelvic ring, the right and left innominates join at the pubic symphysis. Commonly referred to as the pubic "bone," the pubic symphysis is actually a joint made up of *two* bones, one cushioning disc and numerous ligaments. During walking, the pubic symphysis serves as the front axis for the alternating movement of the legs. Similar to the sacroiliac joint, the pubic symphysis helps to decrease pressure within the pelvic ring during walking. Dysfunction at the pubic symphysis alters the mechanics of walking and can cause pain in the groin, inner thighs or abdominal muscles. A misalignment in the pubic symphysis can lead to bladder symptoms such as urgency, frequency and leaking. The pubic symphysis houses the bladder and one of the main PFMs, the pubococcygeus also known as the PC.

The pelvic ring, or pelvic girdle, serves as a transfer station for movement. When we change positions, shift our weight, take a step, or stand on one foot, the weight of our bodies is transferred through the SI joints and pubic symphysis. As explained earlier, the SI joints and pubic symphysis must simultaneously provide stability and allow for motion. For simple activities, such as sitting and standing, most of our stability is provided by the bony architecture of the sacrum fitting tightly in between the two innominates. For more difficult activities, such as walking, stair climbing or running, the tight fit of the SI joints is not enough to stabilize the pelvic girdle. For these demanding activities, the pelvic girdle relies heavily on its muscles and surrounding ligaments.

How Pelvic Alignment Affects the Pelvic Floor Muscles

Optimal pelvic alignment not only affects a woman's ability to move without pain, but alignment also affects the function of the very important pelvic floor muscles. The pelvic floor muscles consist of three layers of muscle that support your pelvis, control urination and defecation and allow for optimal sexual function. Many women become acutely aware of these muscles during pregnancy. Some women experience urinary incontinence due to pelvic floor weakness, while other women experience pelvic pain due to spasm of these very same pelvic muscles. Optimal pelvic floor muscle control can stabilize the low back and pelvis and help prevent incontinence, pelvic pain, and prolapse. Maintaining good pelvic alignment is key to pelvic floor muscle function. The pelvic floor muscles are housed within the bony pelvis and form the secure foundation for pelvic floor muscle contraction and relaxation.

Anatomical Landmarks and Surface Anatomy: The Pubic Symphysis, Anterior Superior Iliac Spine (ASIS), and Posterior Superior Iliac Spine (PSIS)

There are three important bony "landmarks" that we will use to assess your pelvic alignment: the pubic symphysis, the anterior superior iliac spine (ASIS) and the posterior superior iliac spine (PSIS).

Finding the Pubic Symphysis

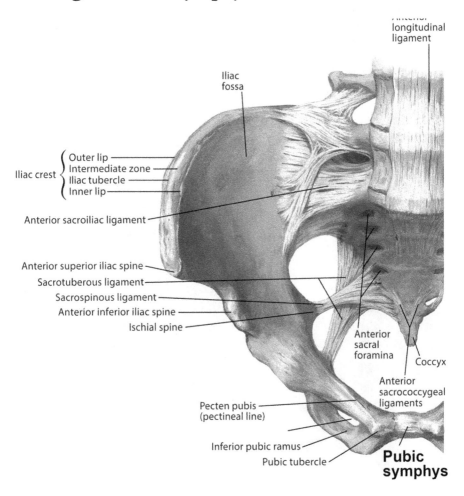

Diagram Description: Notice the pubic symphysis and the ligaments that surround and keep this joint in place. When there is a separation or misalignment of this joint, women experience a great deal of pain and/or suffer from pelvic floor muscle dysfunction and bladder symptoms. Source: Netter Images.

WHAT TO DO:
The pubic symphysis is best located while standing or lying down. Place the heel of one of your hands at your belly button, with your fingers facing down toward your feet until you contact the bones of the pubic symphysis. Remember that the pubic symphysis is actually made up of two separate bones that are joined in the middle.

Finding the Anterior Superior Iliac Spine (ASIS)

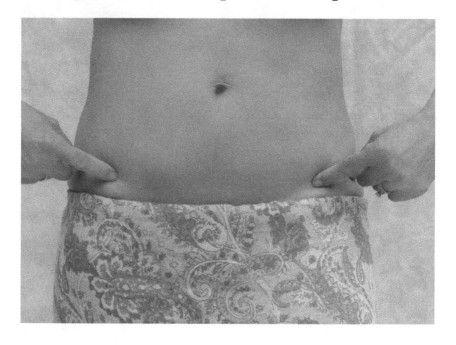

Description: The finger placement shows you the location of the ASIS. You can easily see it in this photograph as this bony prominence sticks out anteriorly. Practice finding ASIS on your body.

WHAT TO DO:
Start by placing your hands on the highest part of your pelvis. Most people naturally assume this position when placing their "hands on their hips." The highest point on your pelvic bones is called your iliac

crest. Now trace your iliac crest forward until you come across two distinct, bony projections toward the front of your pelvis. These two rounded projections are your ASIS.

Finding the Posterior Superior Iliac Spine (PSIS)

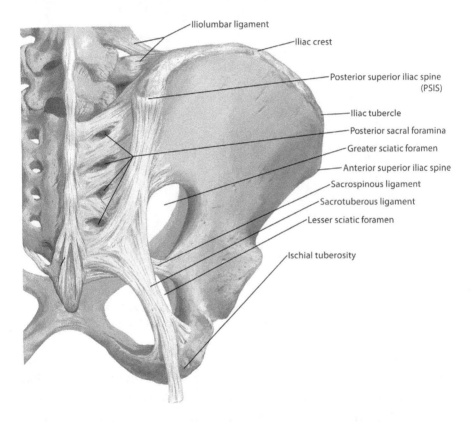

Iliolumbar ligament

Iliac crest

Posterior superior iliac spine (PSIS)

Iliac tubercle

Posterior sacral foramina

Greater sciatic foramen

Anterior superior iliac spine

Sacrospinous ligament

Sacrotuberous ligament

Lesser sciatic foramen

Ischial tuberosity

Diagram Description: Notice the large bony protrusion on the top. That is the PSIS and it can be easily found on most women. Source: Netter Images.

The Dimples of Venus and Their Relationship to PSIS

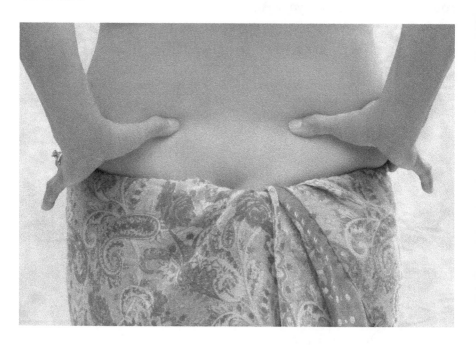

Diagram Description: Notice the indentations on the skin. These dimples are called the "Dimples of Venus" and right next to them you can find the PSIS. The finger location shows you the location of the PSIS.

WHAT TO DO:

Place your hands at the top of your iliac crest. Now trace your iliac crest toward your low back until you come across two rounded bony projections in the low back. These two rounded projections are your PSIS. Some people have small indentations, or dimples, next to their PSIS, making them easier to find. For most people, these are not as easy to find as ASIS.

How to Assess Your Alignment: The Pubic Symphysis

WHAT TO DO:

1. You may be able to directly assess whether the two sides of your pubic symphysis are in alignment. Start by identifying the two bones of your pubic symphysis as described above.

2. Find the very top, or most superior portion, of these bones and slide your thumbs on top of the right and left bone. Now assess whether your thumbs are level, or whether one thumb is higher than the other.

3. If you notice that one side of the pubic symphysis is higher than the other, you may benefit from the shotgun correction described later in this chapter.

4. You may find it difficult to assess the relative heights of the pubic bones but that shouldn't stop you from seeking the help of a friend to access the alignment of the pubic symphysis.

5. If you find an innominate rotation in the next assessment, then you can assume that the pubic symphysis is also out of alignment and you can proceed with the shotgun correction.

How to Assess Your Alignment: Anterior and Posterior Innominate Rotations

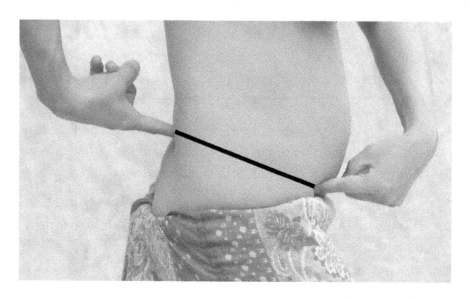

Description: Notice the ASIS and PSIS and the line connecting both. The inclination of this line determines whether you are suffering from a posterior innominate or anterior innominate misalignment. This is normal, optimal alignment.

WHAT TO DO:

1. Stand sideways in a mirror and identify your ASIS and PSIS on your right side. Picture an imaginary line going from your right PSIS to your right ASIS and take note of the angle that this line forms. Although this angle may vary from person to person, the line should slope downward from the PSIS to the ASIS. A recent research article found the average angle from PSIS to ASIS to be thirteen degrees sloped downward from the horizontal.

2. Repeat this procedure on your left side. Take careful notice of whether the line from PSIS to ASIS seems to be sloped more vertical or more horizontal than your right side.

3. If you find that one line is noticeably more horizontal, the innominate on this side may be rotated posteriorly, or backward, compared to the other side. We will refer to this later in the chapter as a posterior innominate.

4. If you find that one line is noticeably more vertical or sloped downward, the innominate on this side may be rotated anteriorly, or forward, compared to the other side. We will refer to this later in the chapter as an anterior innominate.

How to Correct Your Own Alignment Using Muscle Energy Technique (MET)

Muscle energy technique (MET) is a gentle, yet powerful, osteopathic treatment technique. Osteopathic techniques use the hands rather than machinery to diagnose, treat and prevent injury. MET is a specific technique that involves gentle muscle contraction performed against equal resistance in a specific direction. This type of contraction, in which a muscle contracts but does not shorten, is called an isometric contraction.

Muscle energy technique is simple to perform, yet yields powerful results. MET is used to gently mobilize, or move, joints in order to maintain optimal alignment and function. Due to the fact that MET utilizes voluntary muscle contraction, MET also strengthens muscle as it corrects the joint alignment. In addition to mobilizing and strengthening, MET can reduce localized swelling and venous congestion, as muscle contraction helps to "pump" fluid through the lymphatic and venous systems. All of these benefits are derived from a technique that can safely be performed by anyone anywhere.

One of the greatest benefits of using MET is the innate safety of the technique. When performing MET on yourself, you are the one who controls both the muscle contraction and the resistance to the contraction. In this respect, it is the woman who is responsible for the "dosage" of the corrective technique. Since the technique uses a woman's own muscle contraction, the techniques are widely considered to be extremely safe. In the next section, we will explore how to use MET to correct and maintain optimal pelvic girdle alignment throughout your pelvic healing journey.

How to Correct Your Own Pelvis

We will now share five trade secrets with you; while I commonly perform these corrections on my patients, there are a number of low back and pelvic alignment corrections that a woman can safely perform on her body. In order to be your own best healer, you must perform careful investigative work. Your body may need one, two or three of the self-corrections described below. As you move through the following section, perform each alignment assessment and write down your findings. Follow the corrections that are appropriate for your specific findings. Please note that your pelvic alignment may change over the course of days or weeks. Before performing an alignment correction, repeat the appropriate alignment assessment in order to determine the appropriate correction for your body at the specific time.

As you move through the alignment assessments below, you may discover that your body requires more than one alignment correction. In the osteopathic approach to treatment, the specific order that you perform corrections is important to achieving optimal alignment. Once you have identified the specific corrections that you need, refer to the table below for the proper order of the corrections. The lumbar shift and shotgun corrections can be performed as stand-alone corrections. The anterior and posterior innominate corrections should always be preceded by the shotgun correction.

Table 6.1 Trade Secrets: Order of Pelvic Girdle Corrections

1. Lumbar Shift Correction
2. Shotgun Correction
3. *Anterior Innominate Correction
4. *Posterior Innominate Correction
5. *Simultaneous Anterior/Posterior Correction

Anterior and Posterior Innominate Corrections should always be preceded by the Shotgun Correction.

Trade Secret #1: Lumbar Shift Correction

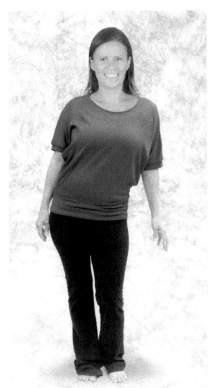

Description: Notice how the upper body shifts away from the lower body. Sometimes a lumbar shift is not this obvious so you really have to scan the body and take notice to determine the shift.

Prior to investigating and correcting dysfunctions of the pelvic girdle, we must first take a quick look at the lumbar spine, or low back region. There are some instances of low back pain and pelvic dysfunction when the upper body shifts away from the lower body in order to take pressure off a painful segment in the low back. It is very important to correct a lumbar shift to avoid further compensation and pain in the low back and legs.

How to Identify

Stand facing a mirror in snug clothing that allows you to see the position of your hips and shoulders. If both of your shoulders are located directly over your hips, then you do not have an obvious lumbar shift and should move on to the next alignment assessment. If you do notice that your shoulders are off to one side when compared to your hips, then you likely have a lumbar shift.

Common Symptoms of Lumbar Shift

A lumbar shift is often seen as a result of back pain that radiates into the buttocks or leg. In many instances, the woman may experience a feeling of tingling or numbness in the leg, rather than pain. Many women report that their leg simply goes weak or collapses under them when they stand up from bed. Some women have no back pain at all, but only symptoms in their leg or foot. All of these symptoms may be due to dysfunction in the low back region. As we mentioned earlier, correcting a lumbar shift is essential to avoid further pain and to enhance PFMs function and strength.

WHAT TO DO:

1.   The motion used to perform the lumbar shift correction is similar to the motion made while playing with a hula hoop or

performing a hula dance. First, make sure to identify your hip position relative to your shoulders, as we are going to slide or "hula" your hips back under your trunk and shoulders.

2. Inhale to prepare for the correction. Exhale and gently engage your transversus abdominis (TrA) as you slide, or hula, your hips back under your shoulders (for instruction on how to properly engage your TrA, see the core chapter). You may also simultaneously slide your shoulders back over your hips. Hold this position and your TrA contraction for five seconds. Then release the contraction and return to your starting position. Repeat the correction ten times.

WHAT TO WATCH OUT FOR:

1. Although you will be shifting into correct alignment, this new positioning may feel very awkward at first, especially if your body has been shifted for a long period of time. Performing this correction over time will help you to regain proper alignment.

2. Performing this correction may cause a brief increase in symptoms. Your symptoms should lessen as you move through the ten repetitions. If your pain increases with repeated repetitions, stop the exercise, as you may not benefit from this correction. You may have a more complex alignment issue and need to be evaluated by a skilled physical therapist.

BENEFITS:

1. Helps PFMs to function optimally yielding a better Kegel-reverse Kegel.

2. Helps to resolve low back pain and sciatica.

3. Helps to strengthen transversus abdominis and maintain spinal alignment.

HOW TO MAINTAIN CORRECTION:

1. Avoid destructive forces to prevent low back pain (see Chapter 5).

2. Abdominal strengthening to stabilize spine (see Chapter 8).

Trade Secret #2: Shotgun Correction for Alignment of Pubic Symphysis

The "shotgun" correction is a pelvic MET that aligns the joint of the pubic symphysis. This is the first correction that is performed if no obvious lumbar shift is noted in the section above. The shotgun correction is appropriate for women who are experiencing bladder symptoms, pubic bone pain, sacroiliac joint pain or PFM dysfunction. Pain at the pubic bone or pubic symphysis is often referred to as symphysis pubis dysfunction (SPD). If you are experiencing symphysis pubis dysfunction, this may be the only correction that you need. If you are experiencing symptoms of sacroiliac joint dysfunction, this will be the first in a series of corrections.

How to Identify

1. Assess your alignment at the pubic bone and innominates as described in the last section.

2. Continue on to the shotgun correction if you find that one side of the pubic symphysis is higher than the other side or if you find an anterior or posterior innominate rotation, as described in the previous section.

Common Symptoms of Symphysis Pubis Dysfunction (SPD)

1. Bladder symptoms, poor Kegel activation, urgency and frequency of urination.

2. Pain in the pubic joint, groin and/or inner thigh with turning over in bed, moving from sitting to standing, walking and going up and down stairs.

3. Inability to stand on one foot while dressing, bathing and/or exercising.

4. Lower abdominal pain, usually greater on one side than the other. The rectus abdominis muscles that form your "six-pack" attach into the pubic symphysis. If the pubic symphysis is in poor alignment, there may be increased tension on these muscles and lower abdominal pain may result and poor activation of your PC muscle.

Shotgun Correction: Phase A (Resistive Abduction) and Phase B (Resistive Adduction)

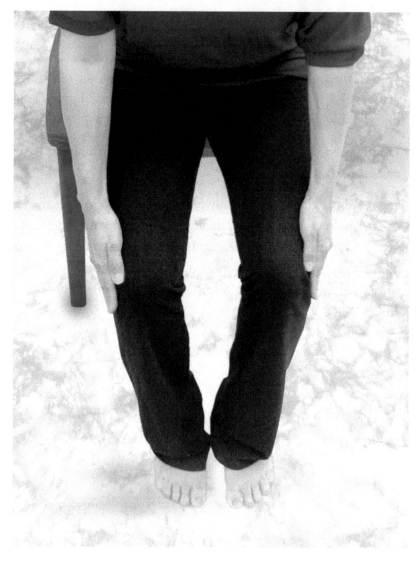

Description: This is called resistive abduction and it's the first phase of the shotgun correction.

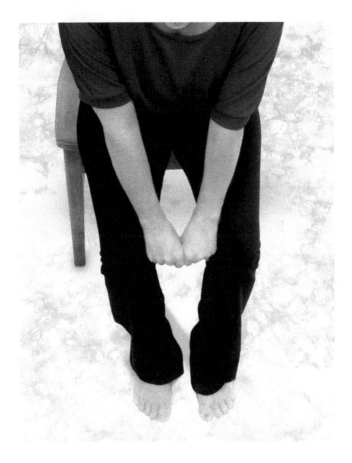

Description: This is called resistive adduction and it's the second phase of the shotgun correction.

WHAT TO DO:

1. This correction can be performed while lying down or sitting up in a chair. A woman can perform the correction on her own or with the help of a partner or friend.

2. If you are seated, scoot toward the edge of the chair and sit up tall. If you are lying down, bend your knees and place your feet flat on the floor or bed. Your knees should be slightly open and in line with your hips and feet.

3. Place your hands on the outside of your knees. While maintaining good posture, if sitting, open the knees and apply resistance to your hands. Press the thighs into your hands as if the legs are trying to rotate away from each other. As the thighs push out into the hands, the hands should apply equal pressure to the thighs, so that the legs do not actually move from their start position. This is called resistive abduction.

4. As you push the thighs into the hands, maintain this contraction for ten seconds. Do not hold your breath during the ten-second contraction. Try to maintain normal breathing, as breath-holding can increase blood pressure and pelvic pressure.

5. Repeat this exercise two more times, for a total of three ten-second contractions.

6. Next, place a firm object between your knees that you can squeeze. You may use a yoga block, firm ball or your own fist. While lying down or sitting in good posture, squeeze your knees against the object for ten seconds. Remember to breathe comfortably throughout the ten seconds. This is called resistive adduction.

7. Repeat the knee squeeze two more times, for a total of three ten-second contractions.

WHAT TO WATCH OUT FOR:

1. In the case of symphysis pubic dysfunction, you may experience pain with the first repetition of the knee squeeze. Ask yourself to rate the pain on a scale of 0 to 10. Then continue to rate your pain during the next two knee squeezes. The pain should

decrease during each repetition. If you are continuing to experience pain with the third repetition, then repeat the ten-second knee squeeze until your pubic pain resolves. In our experience, some women need to perform the knee squeeze up to ten times in order to fully correct the joint alignment, resolve their pain and improve their Kegel activation.

2. It is possible that you may hear a "pop" as the pubic joint corrects into better alignment. This sound is neither dangerous nor necessary for the joint to achieve alignment.

3. If your pain increases, rather than decreases with repeated repetitions, stop the exercise. You may have a more complex alignment issue and need to be evaluated by a skilled physical therapist.

BENEFITS:

1. Helps to resolve bladder symptoms, PFM dysfunction, SPD and sacroiliac joint pain.

2. Strengthening of the inner thigh and outer hip muscles, which are critical to stabilizing your spine and pelvis.

HOW TO MAINTAIN CORRECTION:

1. Avoid destructive forces (Chapter 5).

2. Incorporate abdominal strengthening to stabilize the pelvis (see Chapter 8).

Trade Secret #3: Correction for an Anterior Innominate

How to Identify

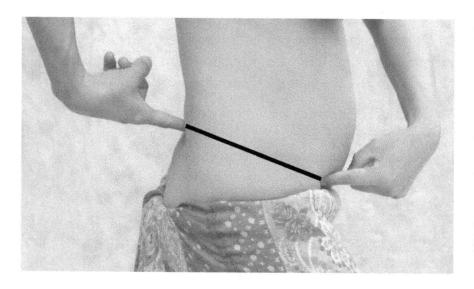

Description: Notice how the ASIS is lower than the PSIS. This is a typical presentation of an Anterior Innominate. Sometimes it's not as obvious as in the photo so you must look very closely.

Using the standing alignment assessment above, identify if one side of the pelvis forms a steeper line when drawn from the PSIS in the back to the ASIS in the front. If you find that one ASIS is significantly lower than the other, and you are experiencing one of the common symptoms listed below, you would likely benefit from an anterior innominate correction.

Common Symptoms of an Anterior Innominate Rotation

1. Pain in the front of the thigh, hip or lower abdomen on the side of the dysfunction.

2. An anterior innominate can also contribute to round ligament pain, which is a sharp, stabbing pain that occurs due to a sudden tightening of a ligament that travels from the uterus to the labia majora.

3. Women with menstrual cramps should check themselves for an Anterior Innominate Rotation.

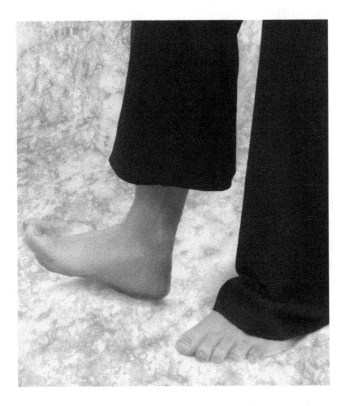

Description: Anterior Innominate correction. Notice the heel digging into the ground. This MET pulls the ilium back from an anterior rotation.

WHAT TO DO:

1. Make sure that you have completed the shotgun correction first and have identified the side of your pelvis that appears to be in an excessive anterior tilt.

2. You may be seated or lying down for this correction. If you are seated, sit toward the front of the chair in good posture. If you are lying down, bend both of your knees so that your feet are on the exercise surface.

3. Press the involved heel down into the floor and hold this isometric contraction for ten seconds. Continue to breathe throughout the contraction.

4. Repeat the ten-second contraction for a total of three repetitions.

WHAT TO WATCH OUT FOR:

1. Do not hold your breath during the contractions, as this may increase your blood pressure.

2. It is best to perform this correction so that the heel presses into a firm surface, such as the floor if performing the correction sitting or a yoga mat if lying down. Some women find that they must perform this correction in bed before rolling to their side to get up. If you are performing this correction on a soft bed, you may be able to modify the correction by clasping your hands behind the involved thigh. You can then press the thigh down into your hands for ten seconds and three repetitions.

3. If, after performing this correction, your pain or symptoms worsen, you may not benefit from this correction. You may have a more complex alignment issue and would benefit from seeing a skilled physical therapist.

BENEFITS:

- Decreased pain with turning in bed, going from sitting to standing and walking.
- Decreased menstrual cramps and better functioning PFMs.
- Strengthening of your hip extensor muscles, including your gluteals, which can help stabilize your spine and pelvis.

HOW TO MAINTAIN CORRECTION:

1. Avoid destructive forces as described in Chapter 5.

2. Incorporate abdominal strengthening to stabilize the pelvis (see Chapter 8).

3. Perform your Kegels regularly.

Trade Secret #4: Correction for a Posterior Innominate How to Identify

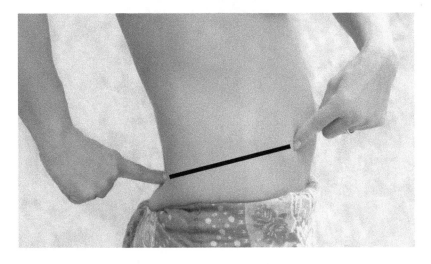

Description: Notice how the PSIS is lower than the ASIS. This is your typical presentation and posterior innominates can contribute to sacroiliac, gluteal and hip pain.

Using the standing alignment assessment above, identify if one side of the pelvis forms a flatter line when drawn from the PSIS in the back to the ASIS in the front. If you find that one PSIS is significantly lower than the other, and you are experiencing one of the common symptoms listed below, then you would likely benefit from a posterior innominate correction.

Common Symptoms of a Posterior Innominate

Pain in the lower back, buttock and/or occasionally pain down the back of the leg on the side of the dysfunction. Many people assume that pain traveling down the back of the leg must be a symptom of a herniated disc; however, a posterior innominate can cause tightness of the piriformis muscle, which can then place pressure on the sciatic nerve.

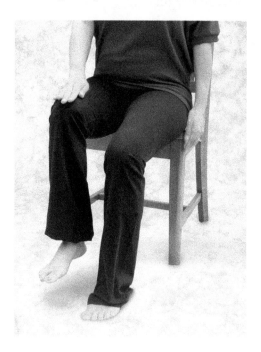

*Description: Notice the hand on the thigh. This MET pulls the ilium
forward from a posterior rotation.*

WHAT TO DO:

1. Make sure that you have completed the shotgun correction first and have identified the side of your pelvis that appears to be in an excessive posterior tilt.

2. You may be seated or lying down for this correction. If you are seated, sit toward the front of the chair in good posture. If you are lying down, bend both of your knees so that your feet are on the exercise surface.

3. Lift the involved knee up to meet your hand. If you are lying down, your knee should form a right angle while in the air. Some women find it difficult to maintain their leg in the air and prefer to start the correction with both legs resting on a ball. Press the involved knee up into your hand. Your elbow should remain locked and your arm should meet your knee with an equal amount of pressure so that the knee does not actually move. Continue to hold this isometric contraction for ten seconds and continue to breathe throughout the contraction.

4. Repeat the ten-second contraction for a total of three repetitions.

WHAT TO WATCH OUT FOR:

1. Do not hold your breath during the contractions, as this may increase your blood pressure.

2. Some women report cramping in the muscles at the front of the hip during this correction. If you experience spasms or cramping of the muscle, decrease the force with which you are pressing the knee into your hand.

3. If, after performing this correction, your pain or symptoms worsen with walking, you may not benefit from this correction. You may have a more complex alignment issue and would benefit from seeing a skilled physical therapist.

BENEFITS:

1. Better PFMs function.

2. Decreased pain with turning in bed, going from sitting to standing and walking.

3. Strengthening of your hip flexor muscles, including the psoas, which can help stabilize your spine and pelvis.

HOW TO MAINTAIN CORRECTION:

1. Avoid destructive forces as described in Chapter 5.

2. Incorporate abdominal strengthening to stabilize the pelvis (see Chapter 8).

3. Perform your Kegels on a regular basis.

Trade Secret #5: Simultaneous Correction of Anterior and Posterior Innominate – Lying Down Simultaneous Correction

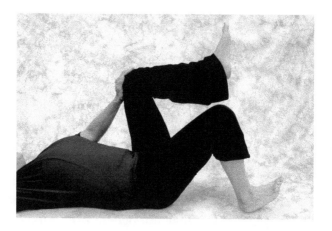

Description: Simultaneous corrections for posterior and anterior innominate can be performed in either a lying down position or seated position.

Seated Simultaneous Correction

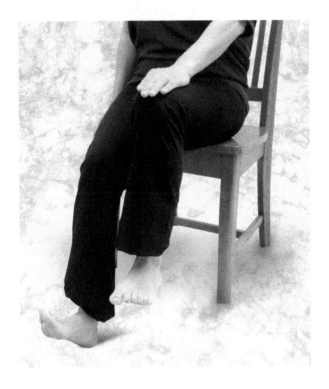

Description: Notice the combination of the heel into the floor to correct an anterior rotation and the thigh press to correct a posterior rotation. They are corrected simultaneously with this seated technique.

As we have just reviewed, anterior innominate correction is appropriate if you find an anterior rotation of the pelvis, while posterior innominate correction is appropriate if you find a posterior rotation of the pelvis. But what happens if you find that you have an anterior rotation on one side, a posterior rotation on the other side, and you do not know which side requires the correction?

Oftentimes, our symptoms will tell us which side is the "dysfunctional" side that requires an MET correction. For instance, if you find a posterior rotation on your left side and you have left low back and buttock pain, then you should perform posterior innominate correction for a left posterior rotation. Along the same line of thinking, if you find an anterior rotation on your right side and you have right hip and groin pain, then you should perform anterior innominate correction for an anterior rotation.

However, if you find an anterior rotation on one side, a posterior rotation on the other side, and you currently do not have pain, or your symptoms are unclear, then you can try a simultaneous correction as described below.

WHAT TO DO:

1. Make sure that you have completed the shotgun correction first and have identified the side of anterior rotation and the side of posterior rotation.

2. You may be seated or lying down for this correction. If you are seated, sit toward the front of the chair in good posture. If you are lying down, bend both of your knees so that your feet are on the exercise surface.

3. On the side of the anterior rotation, press your heel down into the floor. At the same time that you are pressing your heel down on one side, lift the opposite knee (on the side of the anterior rotation) and press the knee up into your hand. Hold both contractions for ten seconds and continue to breathe throughout the contraction.

4. Repeat the simultaneous correction, with one heel pressing down and one heel pressing up two more times, for a total of three repetitions.

WHAT TO WATCH OUT FOR:

1. Do not hold your breath during the contractions, as this may increase your blood pressure.

2. If after performing this correction, your pain or symptoms worsen, you may not benefit from this correction. You may have a more complex alignment issue and would benefit from seeing a skilled physical therapist.

BENEFITS:

1. Better PFM function.

2. Decreased pain with turning in bed, going from sitting to standing and walking.

3. Strengthening of your hip flexor and extensor muscles, which can help stabilize your spine and pelvis.

HOW TO MAINTAIN CORRECTION:

1. Avoid destructive forces as described in Chapter 5.

2. Incorporate abdominal strengthening to stabilize the pelvis (see Chapter 8).

3. Perform your Kegel program regularly.

Beyond the Pubic Symphysis and Innominates: Sacral Torsions

In addition to the pelvic alignment conditions and corrections covered above, there are numerous other spinal and pelvic alignment issues that are beyond the scope of this book. If you are experiencing low back pain that increases with turning over in bed, moving from sitting to standing and walking, and your pain is not relieved with the pelvic corrections prescribed above, you may have a sacral torsion.

A sacral torsion is a rotation of the sacrum that disrupts the normal mechanics of the SI joint. Sacral torsions are often best evaluated and treated in-person by an experienced physical therapist. Make sure to choose a practitioner who has extensive experience treating women with pelvic floor muscle dysfunction.

Now that you know how to correct your own alignment make sure to check it frequently throughout your pelvic rehab program. This self-adjustment is important for the work that comes up in the next chapter dealing with **the right and smart way** to do Kegels. Let's take a look…

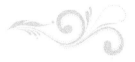

You have come this far, but I have more to teach you.

Untwist the House of Your Pelvic Muscles

…to go deeper ONLINE, visit
http://www.FemalePelvicAlchemy.com/chapter6

Untwisting your pelvic house so your lady parts are happy and in good alignment does not require outside help. In this training video I guide you through a simple correction that is a game-changer; it will help you to restore your erotic power and to keep pain and dysfunction far away and out of your queendom. Check it out—you won't be sorry!

CHAPTER 7

Erotic Power with Alchemical Kegels

We are all in search of the sexual holy grail, but there is very little guidance and just plain old bad information for the goddesses out there. Everywhere I go on social media I see posts about the pelvic floor muscles and their Kegel counterparts that are just wrong. Contrary to popular belief you do not have to lift a surfboard with your vagina, and an overly tight vagina is *not* the goal for your health. Balance is the goal and the path to reclaiming our true goddesses.

The term *Kegel* is used to describe a set of exercises, developed by gynecologist Dr. Arnold Kegel, designed to improve the function of the pelvic floor muscles (PFMs). Typically, Kegels are prescribed for women suffering from incontinence or organ prolapse, and are intended to help strengthen and improve PFM endurance, continence and sexual function by reducing laxity and decreasing weakness. But there are subtle nuances to Kegels that, if not taken into account, can actually produce negative results for women. There is an art to prescribing Kegels and I have finessed this art form by treating thousands of women and helping them to overcome their pelvic and sexual dysfunction. My patients tell me: "My doctor told me to do Kegels; I did and I am still leaking and feeling pressure." Telling women to just do Kegels is not enough; they need to be guided and escorted through this process.

In this chapter I shed light on the topic of Kegels, showing you the right way to start your strengthening Kegel program (also known as uptraining) and how to ensure long-term success. I also cover in great detail the Reverse Kegel (RK). I coined this term 12 years ago when I noticed women were Kegeling themselves into pelvic floor muscle dysfunction. There's a law of physics that states: for every action there is an equal and opposite reaction. Similarly, for every Kegel there is a reverse Kegel, a mindful relaxation of the pelvic floor muscles. Goddesses cannot solely contract their vaginas; they must also be able to "let go and let flow." The action of training your pelvic vaginal muscles to let go is called downtraining. This type of training is for women whose vaginas are too tight and whose pelvic floor muscles have too much tone, spasms or trigger points in them. When the vagina has too much tone, the pelvic floor muscles are hypertonic. When the vagina lacks tone, the pelvic floor muscles are hypotonic. It's possible to have both a hypotonic and hypertonic pelvic floor.

We must keep in mind that the vagina is three-dimensional and not all its parts will be the same. But we can train it to come into balance when it is unbalanced, and this is what you will learn here. You may have thought that all vaginas were loose and relaxed especially after childbirth, but this is not the case at all. This is a media ploy that makes us feel "less than." There is a whole industry out there that relies on the fact that we feel that we are not good enough. This feeling, this way of thinking is about to end.

Women get into trouble with their vaginas when they start to do too much of just one type of training exercise. Your vagina is meant to be supple, flexible, soft yet strong and powerful. If your pelvic floor muscles are too tight, a slew of crazy female issues can arise, issues such as constipation, anorgasmia, deep pelvic ache, hip pain, menstrual cramps, or pain with sex. My point is that balance is a MUST. Balance in your pelvic health program which will include a Kegel and a reverse Kegel in a certain ratio held for a certain amount of time.

Before we get to the nitty-gritty of Alchemical Kegels, you must first understand the pelvic floor muscles, their unique anatomy and function and how to visualize them so you can develop your own training program with my guidance.

Pelvic Floor Muscle Anatomy and Function

The Female Pelvic Alchemy Program begins with understanding your body on an anatomical level, a physiological level, and an energy level. Your pelvic floor is a complex set of muscles, nerves, and connective tissues that can accurately be called the cradle or basket of your being. The PFMs are shaped like a basin, and they are the size of a small salad bowl. On an energy level, the pelvic floor contains the first chakra, or energy center, and supports the other chakras. If the foundation is experiencing stress and trauma, then naturally all of your energy will be affected. Major nerves that innervate your entire lower extremity pass through the pelvic region, and a complex web of muscles and fascia support your uterus, bladder, vagina, rectum, and other abdominal organs. If the muscles in your pelvic floor are in spasm, weak or are filled with trigger points or scar adhesions, your female symptoms will be worse. If your pelvic floor muscles are weak, you can experience sexual dysfunction and a slew of bladder issues including incontinence, urgency and frequency of urination. Many times women will feel as if they cannot completely empty either their bowels or bladders, and they push to get the urine or feces out. Pushing with defecation and urination is a big no-no as this action strains the PFMs and contributes to spasms, trigger points and more weakness.

To understand this area of your body better, we'll take a look at the various constructs of your pelvic floor muscles, also called the levator ani muscles. This is a lot to cover, so remember to consult the extensive glossary as well as to familiarize yourself with key concepts and terms found in this book. By getting to know your own anatomy and its particular nuances, you will find that you can open the door to your own healing and maintain long-term results. You hold the key to turning your goddess power on. Now let's take a look at what I consider to be the most important muscles in the female body—the Pelvic Floor Muscles.

Pelvic Floor Muscles Internal View

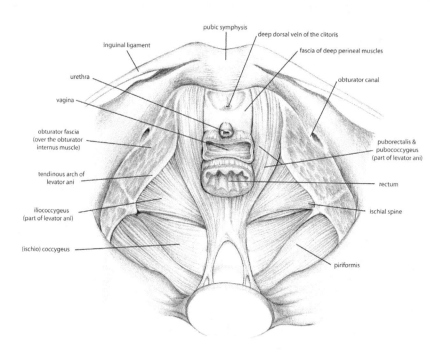

Diagram Description: Top-down view of the pelvic floor. Your body is cut in half at the waist and you are peering down into the third layer of the pelvic floor basket with organs removed. To stretch and work on this layer you need medical clearance from your OB/GYN or midwife. Many times dysfunctions in this third layer cause a deep ache in the vagina, pain with sexual intercourse and pain in the pelvic hip region. Source: Netter Images.

PFMs Functions

The overall pelvic floor muscle group has five primary functions. First, these muscles are supportive and hold your organs up and in place. Second, they are sphincteric and help prevent urinary and fecal incontinence. Third, they are sexual, enhancing and making orgasms stronger. Fourth, they help stabilize the lumbar, sacral, pelvic and hip regions. Fifth, they act like a pump for fluids.

Pelvic Floor Muscles – An Inferior View Highlighting External Genitalia, Perineum, PFM Layer 1, Gluteal Muscles, Levator Ani (PFM Layer 3)

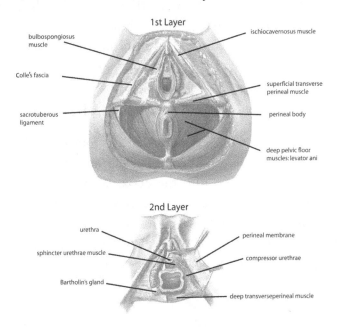

Diagram Description: PFMs first layer appear in the diagram along with some levator ani (third layer PFMs), gluteal muscles. This is the perineal area with the skin removed to reveal the muscles. The first layer is the focal point of stretching during the later part of pregnancy. The first layer is one knuckle deep inside the vagina. This illustration shows the external part of the first PFM layer. Source: Netter Images.

PFMs Innervation

The pelvic floor muscles are innervated by the pudendal nerve, perineal nerve, inferior rectal nerve, the sacral spinal and levator ani nerves. These nerves originate in the low back and tailbone region anatomically known as the L4-S4 region. The muscles of the female pelvic floor can be a source of confusion for many people – even to the trained professional – because they have been given several different names, making it difficult to understand the nomenclature and classification. In this book we will classify the female pelvic muscles into three layers and will describe other structures that must be understood in order to perform vaginal massages. Please look at Table 7.1 for a description of the main muscles and anatomy of the female pelvic floor. Refer to the accompanying anatomy diagrams throughout the chapter as you begin to absorb and understand the techniques I have compiled for the stretching of the perineum. Be scientific in your approach to better visualize the musculature of your own body.

PFMs Layer Description and Visualization

The PFMs can be visualized as a box that has four walls. Think about the walls as an anterior wall, posterior wall and two lateral or side walls. As you move further into the book, keep this visual in mind. The different walls house different muscles, and trigger points in them can reproduce many pelvic and bladder-related symptoms. For instance, if the anterior PFMs are weak and have trigger points and/or muscle spasms and these issues are not resolved, then you can suffer from incontinence, bladder pressure, or urge incontinence. Because the anterior wall of the PFMs houses the uterus and bladder, it is under a lot of stress and should be strengthened with anterior wall Kegels. The anterior wall supports the uterus and the bladder and is found behind the pubic bone which is why the shotgun alignment technique is so important. This technique helps to keep the PFMs and the organs in optimal alignment.

Moving a little deeper into the anatomy of the PFMs, we see that the pelvic floor muscles themselves can be divided into three layers, with each layer progressively deeper inside the vagina. Using your index finger as a road map, the first layer corresponds to the first knuckle, the second layer corresponds to the second knuckle and the deeper layer corresponds to the third knuckle.

Now let's think about the vaginal opening looking like a clock (see diagram below). Twelve o'clock is by the pubic bone, six o'clock by the anus, three o'clock to the left side and nine o'clock to the right. Now imagine that each layer is also its own clock, giving you three clocks, one at each level.

The Clock and Layer Concept

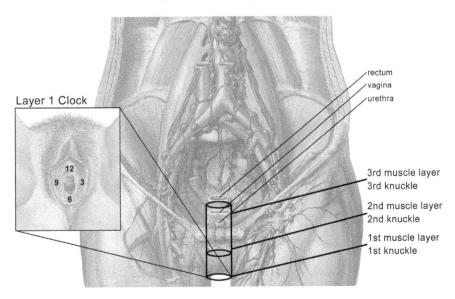

Diagram Description: The PFMs can all be accessed via the vagina. The three pelvic floor muscle layers each correspond to a knuckle of the index finger. The inset shows the clock concept of the first layer. In pregnancy most of the stretching if not all occurs in the first layer of the PFMs to allow the baby's head to go through it.
Source: Netter Images

Table 7.1 Anatomy of Female Pelvic Floor Muscle Layers

Layer Name	Main Muscles	PFM Function
Layer 1 • Located first knuckle of the index finger • Also called urogenital triangle	Bulbospongiosus Ischiocavernosus Superficial transverse perineal muscle External anal sphincter (EAS) External genitalia: includes urethra, lower vagina, vulva, mons pubis, labia majora, labia minora	Sexual
Layer 2 • Located second knuckle of the index finger • Also called urogenital diaphragm	Sphincter urethrae Deep transverse perineal muscle Compressor urethrae muscle Internal anal sphincter (IAS)	Sphincteric
Layer 3 • Located third knuckle of the index finger • Also called pelvic diaphragm	Levator ani: commonly broken down into Pubococcygeus Puborectalis Iliococcygeus Obturator internus Coccygeus	Sexual Supportive Stabilization functions

Now that you have a good idea of the anatomy, function and constructs of the PFMs we will move into our next area: how to do a self-assessment of your PFMs.

Accessing Your Goddess Power: Designing Your Own Pelvic Power Program: How to Access and Start

You will be performing an internal vaginal assessment of the PFMs. This will involve grading your Kegel holding endurance (how long you can hold a Kegel) and your release ability (how long it takes you to release your Kegel completely; also called a reverse Kegel). Perform an internal vaginal examination with your middle finger. You can do this testing in a sitting or side-lying position. In sitting you will place your middle finger into your vagina and in side-lying I like to use the thumb. (Of course, it is also great if your partner can help you here.) During this self-exam you need to find out how many seconds you can hold a contraction, and conversely how many seconds it takes you to release your muscles completely. These two numbers will determine a ratio that you will use as the starting point of your contract/relax or Kegel/reverse Kegel program. For instance, your program could be in a Kegel to reverse Kegel ratio of 1:1; 1:2 or 1:3. (With a 1:1 ratio, you will do a 5-second Kegel and a 5-second reverse Kegel.) Larger ratios are for women who have just graduated from a reverse Kegel program or who have difficulty relaxing their PFMs. Don't rush into a Kegel uptraining program until you have mastered the reverse Kegel. This is important for pelvic floor coordination. Coordination, the ability to contract and to relax the pelvic floor muscles with breath coordination, is another key factor that determines if you have good pelvic health.

How to Determine Your Kegel-Contract/Reverse Kegel-Relax Program Ratio

1. Please have a mirror and lubrication on hand for your exam.

2. Start off by first looking externally at your perineum and performing a contract Kegel.

3. For correct Kegel execution look for the following motions: your clitoris should move slightly downward, your anus should "wink," and the perineal body should move up and in.

4. After looking at your Kegel contraction, look at your reverse Kegel. You should see the anus release and your perineal body move outward toward the mirror.

5. Once you are performing the Kegel and the reverse Kegel correctly, place a well-lubricated index finger into your vagina and contract your PFM around your finger. Count to see how many seconds you can hold the contraction by counting 1 Mississippi, 2 Mississippi, 3 Mississippi, etc. Don't count fast. Count slowly and deliberately. Stop counting once you feel the contraction of the Kegel get weaker or release. This is the number of seconds to use for the contraction.

6. Start releasing your muscles and see how many counts of Mississippi it takes you to release your PFM completely. From these 2 numbers, determine your contract/relax ratio. For example, you might start out with a 5-second Kegel contraction and a 10-second reverse Kegel so your ratio would be 1:2.

7. Always err on the side of safety by giving yourself more time to release. Here's a pearl of wisdom: many women get stuck in the contraction and cannot release their pelvic floor muscles. If this is the case for you, master the reverse Kegel first to be pain free and have somewhat normal tone before attempting Kegels.

Kegel Strengthening Program Contract/Relax or Kegel/Reverse Kegel

1. Now that you have determined your ratio, start your strengthening program conservatively by performing 10 repetitions of contract/relax 1 to 3 times daily, incorporating your ratio as your guide.

2. Pay close attention to make sure your pelvic symptoms do not increase with your current strengthening program. If you start to experience more symptoms, stop the contract/relax exercises immediately and go back to the internal work described previously.

3. After 1 to 2 weeks, if you are doing well with your contract/relax program, start doing your program 3 to 5 times daily. If you have vaginal muscle soreness, skip a day and let your vaginal muscles recover. This is a muscle like any other muscle.

4. After 2 weeks, retest to see if your PFM contract endurance has improved. If it is longer, then add more seconds to your contraction Kegel. For example, if after 2 weeks of diligently doing strengthening exercises, you can now hold your slow Kegels for 7 seconds, then start doing your program with 7 seconds contract and 14 seconds release, using the same 1:2 ratio as a guide. You may find your ratio changes over time, and if so, this is acceptable. The goal for the Female Pelvic Alchemy program is a 1:1 ratio of a 10-second Kegel and a 10-second reverse Kegel (or 2 reverse Kegels which equal 10 seconds).

Quick-Flick Kegels

In conjunction with your Kegel-contract/reverse Kegel-relax program you will add the quick-flick Kegel exercises as well. These consist of 1 to 2 second contracts followed by 1 to 2 second releases, repeated 10 to 20 times. These quick Kegels should be performed after resting for 1 minute after the slow Kegels. For strengthening programs, the goal that I usually set for my patients is a 10-second slow Kegel contraction with a 10 to 20 second release, performed 1 to 5 times daily. After one set of the slow Kegels, I recommend waiting 1 minute and then doing 10 to 20 quick Kegels. By performing both types of Kegel strengthening exercises, you will hit the slow twitch and fast twitch muscle fibers of the pelvic floor. Fast Kegels allow you to brace and pull up pelvic floor muscles before a cough, sneeze or laugh and help you to control leaking. I also recommend quick Kegels for women when they have prolapse or pelvic pressure.

Breathing Counts in the Alchemical Kegel Program

Do not quit if you find yourself feeling frustrated with your breathing and releasing on the inhale. Be content to make small improvements if needed, in the beginning. You will achieve breakthroughs as long as you continue to persevere. Strive for a deep understanding of your body so that you can remain aware of your PFMs with your day-to-day activities.

Log Your Pelvic Assessment Findings Here

1. Determine your ratio (ex: 1:2).

2. Exhale, contract your PFMs for _____ seconds. As you hold the Kegel contraction, breathe naturally or count out loud.

3. Inhale, release your contract, and relax your PFMs for _____ seconds. Imagine you are breathing into your PFMs.

4. The coordination of contract/relax Kegels with the breath is very important for proper execution of the exercise. (For example for 1:2 ratio, exhale as you contract for 3 seconds, inhale and release/reverse Kegel for 6 seconds to ensure full relaxation.) During the relaxation phase, you must consciously release the pelvic floor muscles using your reverse Kegel.

5. Your Recommended Program:
    Beginner: Slow Kegels: 5 second holds; 2 to 3 sets daily; 5 to 10 repetition, using a ____:____ ratio.
    Advance: Slow Kegels: 5 to10 seconds holds: 3 to 5 sets; 10 to 15 repetition, using a ____:____ ratio.

I recommend working up to 20-second Kegels for runners and athletic women who need more power and endurance. For them I advise a big focus on balance with reverse Kegels and stretching of both the upper and lower extremities of their bodies.

Reverse Kegel: The Controversy—Don't Go Any Further Until You Read This

For every action there is a reaction. For every Kegel there must be a reverse Kegel. This is one of the most important laws of pelvic rehab. I find that everyone wants to contract their PFMs but not everyone relaxes the PFMs because women don't know how or have never been taught the correct way to release their PFMs. PFMs that are tight and inflexible will not strengthen. I don't want you to skip this part of your pelvic program. There has to be balance, a yin and yang to your pelvic rehab program. Although the reverse Kegel can be challenging it is not impossible if you have the right guidance.

Let It Go and Let It Flow: Reverse Kegel Muscle Relaxation Series

Your ability to have conscious and mindful release of the pelvic floor muscles is a critical part of your Alchemical Kegel program. The foundation of conscious and mindful release is the mastering of the reverse Kegel relaxation exercise. Your success in your pelvic goddess program relies on your ability to incorporate and do the reverse Kegel correctly. You must learn to focus on and relax these muscles before they can become strong again. Relaxation and lengthening of the PFMs with reverse Kegels is also called downtraining.

The reverse Kegel downtraining series contains three exercises that will help you gain awareness and control over your pelvic floor. At first the PFM relaxation exercises will be extremely difficult to visualize and perform. Many of you have had tension in your lady parts for a very long time. As with anything else, the more you practice these exercises, the easier they will become to do and to implement. Designed to help achieve balance in the PFMs, the reverse Kegel series in this book contains the most effective methods that have brought success to my patients.

The Importance of Breath

To more effectively perform the reverse Kegel series, you must couple the techniques with proper breathing. When I teach my patients the basics of downtraining, I emphasize diaphragmatic breathing to ensure their success. Diaphragmatic breathing can be defined as a type of breathing that involves the abdominal muscles instead of the ribs, shoulders, and neck muscles.

Diaphragmatic Breathing

To practice diaphragmatic breathing, place one hand over your lower belly and one hand at the center of your heart. On the inhale, let your belly gently rise out into your hands, and on the exhale, let the belly flatten. Don't let the breath raise your shoulders, and don't bring your belly in on the inhale and out on the exhale, as this is not diaphragmatic breathing.

The best way to consciously release tension from the PFMs is to do the reverse Kegel while you inhale. Do not be discouraged if you find this difficult to perform. All of my patients have trouble with this concept in the beginning. Just imagine though, that when you inhale properly, your diaphragm actually lowers to make room for the air, so it is natural to also lower and relax the pelvic floor muscles. When you exhale, your diaphragm rises to push the air out, and you can then raise or contract your PFMs and perform your Kegel.

Coordination of Breath with Your Kegel/Reverse Kegel Program

It is important to time your inhalation and exhalation so that they occur over the same length of time. For example, inhale for five seconds, and then exhale for five seconds. I usually recommend to my patients that they inhale for a count of five while consciously dropping and relaxing their PFMs downward. As they contract their PFMs to exhale, they perform the Kegel.

Breathe in for the duration of a reverse Kegel. For instance, inhale for five seconds while simultaneously sending your in-breath to your vagina. I also call this vaginal breathing or goddess breathing. The focus is all on the vagina and opening and letting go. Once the five seconds are over, hold the end point of the reverse Kegel up to three seconds to reaffirm the stretch and to solidify the stretch and release.

Next we will look at some mind/body tools that will help you connect to your reverse Kegel.

Rose Petal Flower Release

WHAT TO DO:

As you breathe in for 5 seconds, send your inhalation breath to your vaginal muscles visualizing and imagining them as a large tight rose flower that is beginning to blossom in the springtime. Imagine the rose opening up petal by petal. Hold the stretch or opening for two seconds. Try this exercise for 5 to 10 breaths.

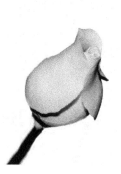 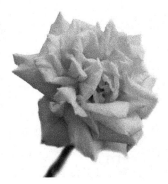

Dropping the Panties

WHAT TO DO:

1. Sit with good posture with your weight evenly distributed on your sit bones.

2. Practice diaphragmatic breathing for several minutes to center yourself.

3. Breathe in for a count of 5 and imagine that your panties and vaginal muscles are dropping into the chair.

4. Make sure to direct your in-breath to your PFMs. With your visualization, collect your pelvic pain and imagine the pain leaving your body with your exhalation or out-breath.

Direct Vaginal Release

WHAT TO DO:

1. Place your clean, gloved finger, vibrator or dilator into your vagina. Try to find a position that is comfortable for you to maintain your finger in your vagina for at least 5 minutes. You can try different positions such as standing, sitting or lying on your side and find the one that works best for you. At times you may be able to do a PFM release in one position but not another. It is important to try all positions to enhance PFM relaxation in any position.

2. As you breathe in, send your in-breath into your vagina and imagine that the walls of your vagina are expanding away from the dilator, vibrator or finger. If you are using a dilator or vibrator you will feel them gently and slowly slip out of the vagina as you do your relaxation exercises.

3. If your dilator/finger is being pushed out as you do your direct release then you are forcing the release and putting undue stress and strain on your pelvic muscles. Pushing to get the release is not the same as gently allowing it to happen with your in-breath. Always couple the visualization with the inhalation.

If you are suffering from sexual pain, pelvic floor muscle tightness, weak orgasms or find yourself gripping your Queendom then you should stay in a Reverse Kegel program until your symptoms improve. Not all goddesses are created equal. Some need to release and let go via a reverse Kegel (downtraining program) before they can even consider doing a contract/relax program.

Cues for Kegels: Mind/Body Connection

The pelvic floor muscles can be difficult to connect with and many women have difficulty doing Kegels the right way. I find that women who use imagery while they do their Kegel exercises get better activation of the pelvic floor muscles and therefore they get more powerful Kegels. Listed below are my top mind/body suggestions; try them all and see which ones work for you. Sometimes placing a finger inside the vagina as you Kegel and use the imagery lets you know which images give you the best PFMs activation. All of this imagery works well for the reverse Kegel as well.

1. Imagine bringing your pubic bone to coccyx as you do your Kegel.

2. Imagine you are stopping the flow of urine.

3. Imagine the vagina is a box with four walls. Bring right wall and left wall together and squeeze. Once you have this squeeze pull the finger up toward your nose.

4. Imagine you are lifting the panties or perineum off the chair as you do your Kegel.

5. Touch your perineal body (the area between your anus and vagina) with your finger and then pull your perineal body away from your finger as you do a Kegel. The perineal body should move up and in. If it moves down toward your finger, you are doing your Kegel incorrectly.

6. Imagine you are picking up a piece of lint off the floor with your vagina as a vacuum cleaner.

7. Imagine you are bringing your sit bones together as you perform your Kegel. Bring the sit bones together and pull upward toward the nose.

8. Imagine you are stopping gas from escaping.

Position for Exercising Your Pelvic Floor Muscles MATTERS

Kegels are an art form and like any art form we need to know the nuances that produce mastery. When starting out with a pelvic health and Kegel program it is best to build upon a strong foundation. The position in which you do your Kegel program matters very much and determines if you will be successful. The different positions have a real purpose and must be chosen with expertise. The effects of gravity must be taken into consideration. The natural progression is to start with easier positions (no gravity) and move to more difficult positions (more gravity).

Table 7.2 Progression of Kegels from Easiest to Most Difficult

Level 1. **Supine-flat on back**: For women who are very weak or whose endurance is below 3 seconds and are having difficulty performing their Kegel program. This position eliminates the effects of gravity and is the easiest position for performing your Kegel exercises.
Level 2. **Resting position:** Helps women who suffer from organ prolapse or are experiencing a lot of pelvic pressure either throughout the day or at the end of the day. This position is also great for women with a lot of pelvic weakness. The resting position allows for gravity to assist bladder/uterus back to its normal position so that the contraction can be more effective.
Level 3. **Semi-recumbent:** In this position you are sitting but leaning back supported by pillows. It is between upright sitting and lying down.
Level 4. **Sitting:** Upright sitting makes Kegels more challenging but not as difficult as standing.
Level 5. **Standing:** This position is for women who are advanced and can maintain at least a 5-second Kegel.

Level 6. **Squat plié:** This is a motion Kegel and trains the muscles to work efficiently when you are moving or changing positions. This type of Kegel is very challenging.
Level 7. **Squat exercise:** This is also a motion Kegel and trains the pelvic floor muscles to work more efficiently and to strengthen.
Level 8. **Functional/impact activities such as running**: Kegels while you are doing a certain type of activity that caused or increased symptoms.

To ensure success it is advisable to start out in the easiest position and then progress to more difficult positions. Once you can do three good sets of a Kegel in a certain position you can progress to the next. Many times you can be "in between" positions so you can do two sets at a lower positional level and one set at the next more difficult level. The goal is to strengthen your muscles in the position where you are most symptomatic. Most women experience leaking or pressure in upright positions so it is important to train your muscles in these more advanced positions to ensure success with the program.

So Many Kegels, So Little Time
Table 7.3 Alchemical Kegels from Easiest to More Advanced

Supine Kegels: Slow and Quick
Semi-Reclined Kegels: Slow and Quick
Seated Overflow Adduction: Inner Thigh
Seated Overflow Abduction: Outer Thigh
Seated Combo Kegels: Can be done standing
Seated Down Elevator Kegel: Can be done standing

Standing—Squat Plié
Standing—The Leaning Goddess
Standing—Tree Pose Kegel
Standing—Flipster Kegel
On Ball or sturdy chair: Prolapse Internal Rotations with band
On Ball or sturdy chair: Prolapse External Rotations with band

Alchemical Trade Secret: Supine Kegels

This is the easiest position to do your Kegels, but you must be careful with your body positioning. My recommendation is that you build your endurance to at least 5 seconds before you attempt the seated Kegels. But don't waste too much time in the supine position because most of us have no pelvic floor issues when we are lying down in bed. You want to set yourself up for success, so don't rush it—but don't go too slow either! Many times when I am lying down at night I still perform supine Kegels. You can also do the overflow Kegels in supine. Performing the overflow Kegels hook-lying with knees bent and a resistance band around your thighs helps to improve your pelvic power very quickly. When using a resistance band always start with the easiest resistance and then progress from there. Resistance bands come in different colors that correspond to how much resistance they provide when in use. Start with light resistance and then go to more difficult resistance when you feel you are ready.

Goddess Effect: Helps to improve pelvic floor muscle power, endurance and coordination without the effects of gravity. This would be ideal for a goddess who is just starting out and is very weak or whose endurance is less than 5 seconds. I still do these when I've had a very busy day and I'm tired. I rather that you do something than nothing at all.

Alchemical Trade Secret: Semi-Relined Kegels

After supine or hook-lying, perform your Kegels in a semi-reclined position, with some pillows behind your back. This position is challenging but not as challenging as sitting upright. Again you can place a band around your thigh and do the overflow Kegels as explained below. Overflow in the semi-reclined position produces quick results. (Plus you can do them in bed.) When using a resistance band always start with the easiest resistance.

Goddess Effect: This position prepares you for the more challenging seated and standing Kegels. Practicing your Kegel/reverse Kegel program in this position sets you up for success and helps you to connect with your vagina. I like to do these in bed with my vaginal weights when I am reading at night.

Alchemical Trade Secret: Seated Overflow Kegels

One of my favorite Kegels to prescribe is the overflow Kegel. This Kegel works on the principle that a strong muscle will help a weaker muscle to get strong. The PFMs have fascial connections to the thigh muscles. In the overflow Kegel we use the inner thigh and outer thigh muscles to help the PFMs improve their strength and endurance.

Alchemical Trade Secret: Overflow Kegel— Seated Adduction

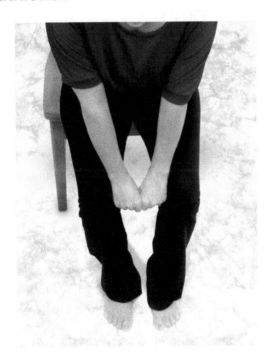

WHAT TO DO:

1. Sit on a stable surface with your feet flat on the floor, hip-width apart, in neutral spine.

2. Make a fist with one or both hands, and place them between your knees. You may also use a pillow or yoga block placed between the knees if you have difficulty maintaining neutral spine while reaching forward.

3. Do a transverse belly hold, Kegel and simultaneously squeeze your fists or pillow/block. This should be an isometric contraction, meaning the legs should not move while you're squeezing.

4. Hold for five seconds and repeat ten times. Do one to three times per day.

WHAT TO WATCH OUT FOR:

1. Holding the breath, which can increase abdominal pressure and cause leaking, pain, and pressure.

2. Rounding your back when you place your hands inside your knees. You must maintain neutral spine to protect your back.

3. You could experience some pubic bone pain with this Kegel and that could mean that your pubic bone is misaligned. Make sure to correct this bone using the tools in Chapter 6, **Untwist the House of Your Pelvic Muscles**.

Goddess Effect:

1. Strengthens the first layer of the pelvic floor muscles, the sexual layer that will help improve orgasms and pelvic power.

2. Helps to keep the bladder and uterus in their optimal place.

3. Has a global effect on all the layers of the pelvic floor muscles by creating an overflow effect. Basically we are using a strong muscle (inner thigh) to get the pelvic floor muscles to fire up and work more effectively. This is a super powerful exercise when you are trying to get stronger faster.

4. Helps to maintain optimal alignment for the lumbar, pelvic, hip and sacral bones.

Alchemical Trade Secret: Overflow Kegel-Seated Abduction

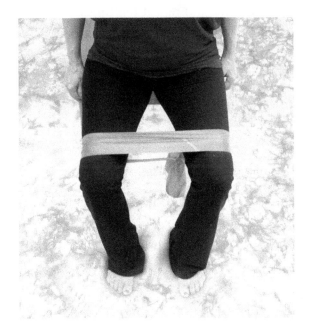

WHAT TO DO:

1. Sit on a stable surface with your feet flat on the floor, hip-width apart, in neutral spine.

2. Place your hands on the outside of your thighs just above your knees. Or if you have a Dyna-Band, you can place it around both thighs just above the knees.

3. Do a transverse belly hold, Kegel and simultaneously push both legs out against your hands or against a resistance band. This should be an isometric contraction, meaning the legs should not move as you push them into your hands or when you press your thighs into a band.

4. When using a resistance band always start with the easiest resistance.

5. Hold for five seconds and repeat ten times. Do one to three times per day.

WHAT TO WATCH OUT FOR:

1. Holding the breath, which can increase abdominal pressure and cause leaking, pain, and pressure.

2. Rounding your back when you place your hands next to your knees. You must maintain neutral spine to protect your back.

3. Pushing your legs out with too much force. Ensure your legs stay stable as you push them into your hands. If you are working with a Dyna-Band move your thighs against the band.

Goddess Effect:

1. Strengthens the third and deepest layer of the pelvic floor muscles.

2. Strengthens the gluteal muscles in particular the gluteus medius which is a primary stabilizer of the pelvic region and helps you to stay pain free.

3. Strengthens PFMs quickly using the overflow effect thereby improving continence, pelvic pressure, organ prolapse symptoms and sexual function.

4. Has a global strengthening effect on all your lady muscles.

Alchemical Trade Secret: Advanced Kegels Combination and Elevator Kegels

The following exercises will help further strengthen and challenge your pelvic floor muscles. This special type of training will increase your strength and endurance for proper bladder and bowel control as well as pelvic organ support and core stability.

Alchemical Trade Secret: Combination Kegel – (Slow Kegel + Quick Flicks)

WHAT TO DO:

1. Squeeze your pelvic floor muscles and continue to hold them for 5 seconds, then build on that contraction by 3 to 4 quick flicks (of your maximal contraction). The entire contraction should last 10 seconds, with a 10-second relaxation between each effort.

2. Repeat this exercise 1-3 times per day. Once you have mastered the exercise while sitting, perform this Kegel while standing.

WHAT TO WATCH OUT FOR:
Holding the breath, which can increase abdominal pressure and cause leaking, pain, and pressure.

Goddess Effect:

1. The combo Kegel is a game-changer. It pulls all the wisdom of the alchemical Kegel program together giving you even more power and endurance and improved coordination.

2. This particular Kegel helps to improve your endurance when you are not progressing and you are stuck at a particular number of seconds.

3. It can be done in a seated or standing position and even in a flat lying down position when you are having trouble improving your power.

4. This Kegel affects all three layers of the PFMs.

Alchemical Trade Secret: THE DOWN ELEVATOR KEGEL

WHAT TO DO:

1. Squeeze your pelvic floor muscles (Kegel exercise) maximally and continue to hold them for 5 seconds, then partially relax and hold at that level for 1 second, then partially relax and hold at that level for 1, then partially relax and hold at that level for 1, then partially relax and hold at that level for 1, then partially relax and hold at that level for 1, and then relax completely.

2. Imagine that your vagina is an elevator stopping at 4 different floors for one second. The whole exercise should take 10 seconds: 5 second hold at the top and 5 small releases on each floor.

3. Repeat this exercise 1-3 times per day.

4. Once you have mastered the exercise while sitting, perform this Kegel while standing.

WHAT TO WATCH OUT FOR:
Holding the breath, which can increase abdominal pressure and cause leaking, pain, and pressure.

Goddess Effect:

1. The down elevator Kegel is all about improving coordination and power.

2. This Kegel works the PFMs improving their strength quickly. It can be difficult to do but the rewards are amazing.

3. It can be done in a seated standing position and even in a flat lying down position.

4. This Kegel works all the layers of the pelvic floor muscles and helps you to train your PFMs for sex because they help you to open up.

Standing Kegels

This is the final frontier for the Emerging Goddess pelvic program. You should be strong enough to do Kegels in the standing position. Don't rush to get here. You can always mix and match levels. For instance, you could do one set of Kegels standing and two sitting.

Alchemical Trade Secret: Squat Plié Kegel

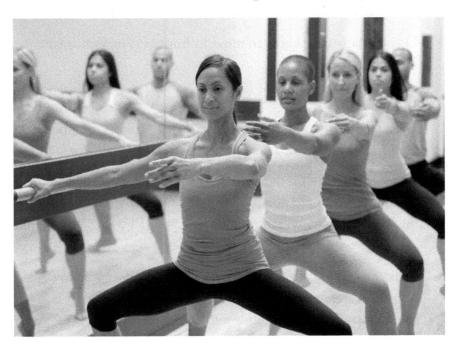

WHAT TO DO:

1. Turn your toes out so that your hips are externally rotated as in ballet position.

2. Bend your knees and lower into a squat plié position.

3. Perform a Kegel for the recommended length of time while you hold the squat plié.

4. Reverse Kegel as you resume standing position.

5. Repeat 10 times; perform 3 sets.

WHAT TO WATCH OUT FOR:

1. Holding your breath, which can increase abdominal pressure and cause leaking, pain, and pressure.

2. Excessive arching or rounding of your back when you lower into your squat – maintain lumbar spine in neutral position.

3. Do not allow your knees to move in front of your toes as you lower into the squat.

Goddess Effect:

1. The squat plié Kegel is a power Kegel that allows all the pelvic floor muscles to work against the full strength of gravity.

2. This Kegel allows for dynamic stretching of the PFMs. You could just go up and down during this exercise without holding the Kegel and you will in essence train your PFMs to be dynamic and more responsive.

3. Squat plié helps to train the muscles to deal better with prolapsed organs—uterus, bladder or rectum—because it is training you in the position where you are the most symptomatic.

Alchemical Trade Secret: The Leaning Goddess

WHAT TO DO:

1. Lean forward from your ankles so they're in a flexed position; allow your body weight to rest on a wall or high table in front of you.

2. Do a transverse belly hold, Kegel and hold the Kegel for the recommended length of time while you hold this plank position.

3. For extra connection place one finger on your urethra (the hole where your urine comes from) and think that you are closing off this hole by contracting the muscles that surround it. This is the second layer of the PFMs.

4. Reverse Kegel as you resume standing position.

5. Repeat 10 times; perform 3 sets.

WHAT TO WATCH OUT FOR:

1. Holding your breath, which can increase abdominal pressure and cause leaking, pain, and pressure.

2. Make sure the flexion comes from your ankles and not from your hips.

Goddess Effect:

1. Strengthens the pelvic floor muscles in a weight-bearing position.

2. Strengthens the anterior wall where the bladder and uterus live and the second layer of the PFMs thereby improving continence, pelvic pressure, organ prolapse symptoms and sexual function.

3. If you are leaking or feeling pelvic pressure due to a bladder or uterine prolapse then this Kegel is for you and will help you to stay dry and improve your continence.

4. If standing is too difficult then do this Kegel in seated position and lean forward. You will make contact with your urethra, the opening where urine comes out from. When you perform this Kegel in a seated position, imagine you are contracting your urethra.

5. Improves goddess power and helps to enhance your orgasms.

Alchemical Trade Secret: Standing Tree Pose Kegel

WHAT TO DO:

1. Balance on your left leg and pick up your right foot and place it on the inner part of your left leg, just below your knee (tree pose).

2. After you get into position do a transverse belly hold, Kegel for the recommended length of time while you hold tree pose. For extra overflow gently press your right foot into the leg. This activates the inner thigh muscles and creates an overflow into the PFMs.

3. Reverse Kegel as you resume standing position.

4. Repeat on the opposite leg. Repeat 10 times; perform 3 sets.

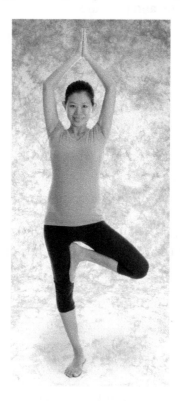

WHAT TO WATCH OUT FOR:

1. Holding your breath, which can increase abdominal pressure and cause leaking, pain, and pressure.

2. Do not let your lifted leg rest on the knee of your balancing leg as this may cause injury to your knee joint.

Goddess Effect:

1. Strengthens the right and left PFMs. Remember that your vagina is three dimensional and we cannot ignore the left and right walls of the vagina.

2. Strengthens the pelvic floor muscles in a weight-bearing position by using the overflow principle.

3. Improves balance and tones the legs while connecting and grounding you to the earth's energy.

4. Strengthens the gluteal and hip muscles.

5. Improves continence, pelvic pressure, organ prolapse symptoms and sexual function.

6. Improves goddess power and helps to enhance your orgasms.

Alchemical Trade Secret: Standing Flipster

WHAT TO DO:

1. Stand with legs hip-width apart in excellent posture with knees slightly bent.

2. Do a transverse belly hold, Kegel and simultaneously press the outer part of your feet into the floor.

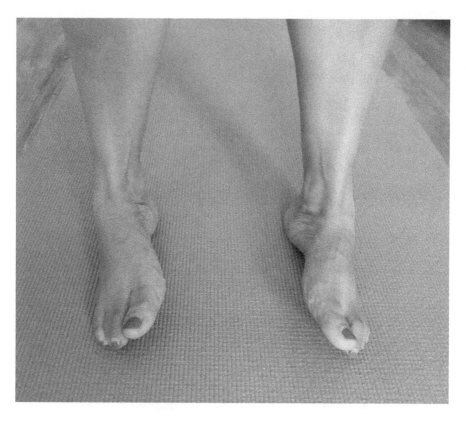

WHAT TO WATCH OUT FOR:

1. Holding your breath, which can increase abdominal pressure and cause leaking, pain, and pressure.

2. Be careful with putting too much pressure and rolling over and twisting your ankle.

Goddess Effect:

1. Strengthens the pelvic floor muscles in a weight-bearing position and helps to improve the function of the right and left PFMs.

2. Strengthens the gluteal and hip muscles and the obturator internus (OI). The OI is a muscle that contains the pudendal artery, nerve and vein. Although this is not a pelvic floor muscle, it can be found within the vagina at the right and left walls. It is important to keep this muscle strong yet supple. When this muscle becomes too tight it can create all kinds of pelvic problems and contribute to pain. This is not a Kegel that should be overused; use it in a way that makes sense and doesn't increase your symptoms or pain.

3. Strengthens PFMs using the overflow principle, improving pelvic power very quickly and helps to maintain pelvic alignment.

4. Athletic women, runners and high impact athletes will benefit greatly from adding this Kegel into their programs. Make sure to stretch your hips out after you do this Kegel so that you don't become too tight in the vagina.

When the Queen Has Fallen, She Needs Help: Prolapse Kegels
Hip Internal Rotation Prolapse Kegel

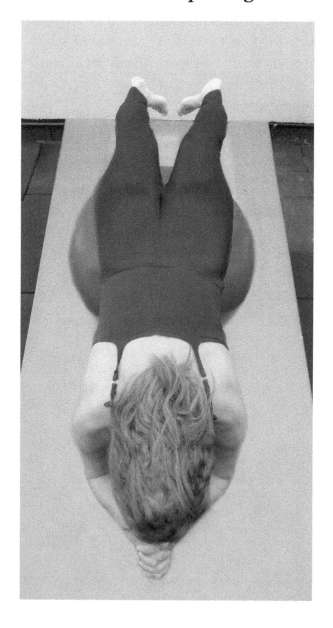

WHAT TO DO:

1. Lying prone on a ball or stool with a resistance band around your legs, turn your toes in toward each other to internally rotate your hips. Perform a Kegel for the recommended length of time while you hold the position.

2. Reverse Kegel as you resume a neutral hip position.

3. Repeat 10 times; perform 3 sets.

WHAT TO WATCH OUT FOR:

Holding your breath, which can increase abdominal pressure, leaking and pain.

Goddess Effect:

1. Reduces stress on the pelvic floor muscles by getting the organs in a better position. In this position the organs move back into a central location and the PFMs can be strengthened more effectively.

2. Use a resistance band around your ankles to improve power more quickly and easily and to help reduce the sensations and discomfort of pelvic pressure and prolapsed organs.

3. The Toes-In position helps to strengthen the anterior wall improving the positioning of the bladder and uterus. Helps to improve vaginal flatulence or "Varts," which are common in women who have PFM weakness.

4. Strengthens all layers of PFMs thereby improving continence, pelvic pressure, organ prolapse symptoms and sexual function.

Prolapse Kegel
Hip External Rotation Prolapse Kegel

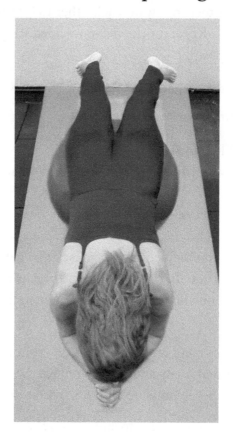

WHAT TO DO:

1. Lying prone on a ball or stool with a resistance band around your legs, turn your toes out to externally rotate your hips.

2. Perform a Kegel for the recommended length of time while you hold the position.

3. Reverse Kegel as you resume a neutral hip position.

4. Repeat 10 times; perform 3 sets.

WHAT TO WATCH OUT FOR:

Holding your breath, which can increase abdominal pressure, leaking and pain.

Goddess Effect:

1. Reduces stress on the PFMs by getting the organs in a better position with a focus on the rectum. Many women suffer from rectal prolapse and this Kegel definitely helps to minimize effects of a rectocele (rectal prolapse).

2. Use a resistance band around your ankles to improve power more quickly and easily and to help reduce the sensations and pressure you may be feeling in your vagina or anus.

3. The Toes-Out position helps to strengthen the posterior wall improving the positioning of the rectum. Helps to improve anal flatulence or air escaping from the anus, which is common in women who have PFM weakness.

4. Strengthens all layers of PFMs thereby improving continence, pelvic pressure, organ prolapse symptoms and sexual function.

Here are some **sample** pelvic health programs. Note that you can do them all lying down, seated or standing or mix and match depending on what's giving you the best results.

Sample Pelvic Health 1

- Reverse Kegel program only 3 to 5 times daily or hourly if there's a painful flare-up.

Sample Pelvic Health 2

- Seated Overflow with inner thigh and appropriate Reverse Kegels: AM session.
- Seated Overflow Out Thigh: PM session
- Prolapse Kegel Toes-In: evening session

Sample Pelvic Health 3

- Squat Plié Kegel
- Elevator Kegel
- Tree Pose Kegel

Goddesses Need Their Massages
Internal PFM-Vaginal Massaging and Stretching Techniques for Balance, Increased Sensuality and Pelvic Power

Vaginal clock stretching and vaginal strumming are internal vaginal techniques that stretch and help improve PFM flexibility, balance, strength and sexual function. Internal massages also help to improve sensation, strengthen orgasms, normalize tone and reduce tension and pain. Although perineal massage is widely known, many women are confused about how to do internal vaginal massages. This upcoming section will bring clarity to these vaginal massages, which are as important to our health as the air that we breathe. Vaginal massage and stretching is suggested for healthy and well-nourished women who wish to improve and create balance in their pelvic muscles. Vaginal massage is amazing for women who tend to be tight in their PFMs or who have difficulty with reverse Kegels.

I find that many women will need to try different body positions such as side-lying or sitting back to make the vaginal stretching techniques comfortable. Additionally, you may have to use your right hand to stretch the left side of the PFMs and left hand to stretch the right side of the PFMs. The most important thing is to try. The more flexible your PFMs are the more easily you will be able to strengthen them. Vaginal muscles that are tight and inflexible will not strengthen easily no matter how many hundreds of Kegels you perform. This is the primary reason why I am introducing this concept of vaginal stretching here. I find too many women doing way too many Kegels without incorporating the balance of pelvic stretching and the reverse Kegel exercises. Balance is very important in a pelvic health program and should not be overlooked. Additionally massaging your vaginal muscles can lead to releasing long-held tensions and trauma. Don't be surprised at how vulnerable you may feel after you massage yourself. Many of my patients cry and many others retrieve memories they had long forgotten. There is an energy to these magnificent massages that benefits many women in their pelvic programs. Don't be afraid to try them and don't be afraid that you will stretch yourself too much. This is a mind game that has been played on us for years. Our vaginas are lovely. They are not overstretched or too big. Through these exercises you will be able to restore balance and tone and everything else in between. **Long live the Queen!!!**

Keeping the Queen Flexible with Internal Stretching

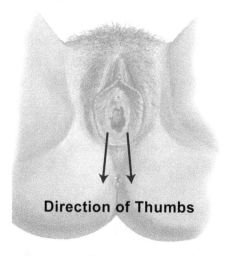

Direction of Thumbs

Diagram Description: The arrows represent the direction of the stretching. The stretching pressure is downward toward the rectum. Do this at the first layer only. Source: Netter Images.

WHAT TO DO:

1. Lubricate your thumbs, insert them into the vagina up to the first knuckle, and press straight downward toward the rectum for three to five minutes.

2. After three to five minutes, press down to the right for several seconds and then to the left for several seconds.

3. If you've recently had a baby you must be completely healed in the perineum before attempting this stretch or any other internal stretching.

4. This stretch helps to soften scar tissue, increase sensation and normalize tension and/or pain.

Pelvic Floor Muscle Vaginal Clock Stretching: All Layers

The pelvic floor muscle clock stretching technique works great for women who have pain with initial penetration, painful scars, or spasms in their muscles. This PFM clock stretch is more specific and stretches the layers of the PFMs in a more well-rounded way. With traditional perineal massage the PFMs are stretched at the 6 o'clock spot but with the clock stretch we are focusing on the lower half of the PFMs. For this method, imagine again that your vaginal opening is a clock. To review, 12 o'clock is by the clitoris, 6 o'clock is by the rectum, 3 o'clock is to the left and 9 o'clock is to the right. Using your finger, start stretching your vagina with the clock as visualization. Remember that the PFMs are divided into three layers, each layer corresponding to the knuckles of the finger and progressively deeper inside the vagina. The first PFM layer is knuckle one, the second PFM layer is knuckle two, and the third PFM layer is knuckle three. For this technique you are focusing on all three layers or just the first layer.

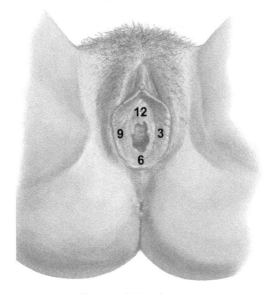

Source: Netter Images.

WHAT TO DO:

Focus your stretching from 4 to 8 o'clock positions, avoiding 12 o'clock where the bladder is located.

1. Insert your finger into the vagina up to the first knuckle only and stretch PFM layer one only. Then insert your finger to the second knuckle and stretch the second layer. Then proceed to the third layer.

2. Press around the clock for thirty to sixty seconds or until you feel a release in the vaginal muscles. You can go around the clock two to three times or you can stay on the same spot for one to three repetitions of thirty to sixty seconds.

3. Only use lubricants that are organic, alcohol free, and paraben free.

4. This stretch helps alleviate pain, trigger points or high tone in the vaginal muscles. Note that if you come across pain, press into it for up to 90 seconds. Do so respectfully and within your pain threshold. When you hold the painful spot it should be getting better not worse. You should not experience any tingling nerve pain or numbing when you are on a spot. If you experience this, you are probably on a nerve or artery and you should get off that spot.

Internal Pelvic Floor Muscle Half-Moon Strumming Massage

Strumming improves the flexibility of the PFMs so they can maximally contract and relax at will. This method involves all three layers of the PFMs.

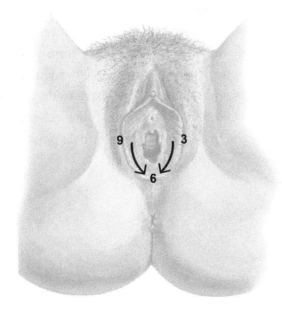

Source: Netter Images.

WHAT TO DO:

1. Strumming massage is a type of massage that is performed in the direction of the pelvic floor muscle fiber. So this massage is from superior to inferior, or top to bottom.

2. Insert your finger (index or thumb) into the vagina up to the first knuckle. First strum the right half of the PFM and then strum the left half, massaging layers 1 to 3 of the PFMs. This massage helps us to connect to our sexual power and is part of every goddess's self-care program.

3. Massage the left half from the 3 to 6 o'clock positions for up to one minute. Rest. Switch hands; massage the right half from the 9 to 6 o'clock positions for up to one minute.

4. Try different body positions such as side-lying or sitting back to make these techniques comfortable.

The techniques and exercises found in this chapter will arm you with some very powerful tools that can help you reclaim the goddess within you. Read all the sections carefully before doing any of the exercises in this chapter. Then go to it! Be confident and know that you have the answers within you. All you have to do is listen carefully to your inner voice when it speaks to you. Now let's move to the next step: core work for the restoration of your female power.

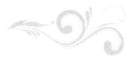

You have come this far, but I have more to teach you.

Erotic Power with Alchemical Kegels

...to go deeper ONLINE, visit
http://www.FemalePelvicAlchemy.com/chapter7

Pelvic and sexual power is the holy grail we are seeking. We search for this because we look for ways to connect with ourselves and with others—especially our lovers/partners. In this video I will help you to understand how to care for your lady parts in a way that you have never before envisioned. Go get this training and forever be changed.

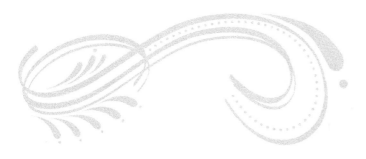

CHAPTER 8

The Truth About Training Your Abdominal Muscles

We are so fixated on what our abs look like that we are willing to try almost any new fad workout or diet that's on the market today. Women in general judge themselves too harshly if they don't have a perfect-looking midsection. I recently treated a woman with what I thought were perfect abs and she still complained about the fat on them. I saw only beauty. I find that most women train their abs incorrectly, using traditional crunches, holding their breath and pushing so hard that they are actually exercising themselves into sexual and pelvic dysfunction. Here's the truth: pretty abs do not make the goddess. Pretty abs do not even create function and sexual power. The fact is that when you train the core properly (without the hype that magazines and the media push on us) your abs will not only look amazing but they will serve to protect your lady parts, your whole pelvic area and your energetic system.

Our abdominal muscles serve a far greater purpose than looking tight and awesome. This area is part of what I call the Pelvic Power relay station. The abdominal muscles create stability in our hips, PFMs and lumbar spine. Our midsections also provide support and stability for our internal organs, house the first two chakras and prevent energy leaks. If your abdominals are in a weakened state or are compromised by having a diastasis recti separation, you are at greater risk for female-related pelvic dysfunction. These problems include an increase in urinary leaking, urgency and frequency of urination, sexual dysfunction, abdominal trigger points, pelvic floor muscle weakness or spasms, pelvic/low back pain and weak or non-existent orgasms. It's important to note here that our abdominal muscles are connected to our pelvic floor vaginal muscles via the fascial system. Fascia is the glue or connective tissue that holds everything together and allows communication between our various systems, organs and muscles.

I cannot overstress the importance of intelligent core training. Many goddesses love to work their abdominals, but are doing it all wrong by performing outdated exercises such as traditional crunches. Performing the same old crunches will not improve your female pelvic power. In fact, traditional abdominal exercises can actually be contributing to your female pelvic symptoms and reducing your goddess effect.

Women who have undergone abdominal surgeries, Cesarean births and myomectomies must really focus on properly re-training their core in order to prevent the incontinence, pelvic pain and muscle spasms that are so prevalent after surgery. For women with pelvic pain, the core is not something to be ignored. Women with pelvic pain are often told not to work on their abdominals because they risk having more pain. Sensible and intelligent core training will help women with both PFM weakness and spasms.

The exercises in this chapter do not require that you put your hands behind your head and lift your shoulders off of the floor. Instead you will be working on the deepest abdominal muscle, the transversus abdominis, while simultaneously engaging your PFMs. This co-contraction creates power from within the body and can result in lifelong changes to your pelvic function. Proper co-contraction can result in improved sexual power, better bladder and bowel control, and less pelvic pain.

This co-contraction is a low-level gentle contraction of the PFMs and the transversus abdominis. Co-activation is not about gripping the PFMs nor is it about pulling in the abdominals with too much force. If you over-contract your core and focus only on the pretty lines of the external oblique abdominal muscles and the six-pack muscles of the rectus, you risk certain dangers. When we train only our external abdominal muscles and create too much tension in them, we create what I call a piston effect during the exercises. This piston effect creates intra-abdominal pressure, muscle tension and can increase your risk of organ prolapse and leaking. You've probably heard the stories: "I worked my core so hard that I peed on myself" or "Every time I do a crunch I orgasm." Although I love my orgasms, I don't think it's a good idea to "come" when you are working out.

When you co-contract the PFMs and the transversus abdominis you do it at about 20 to 30 percent effort. This is a gentle effort that creates a root-lock mechanism, the kind all the yogis are talking about. The synergistic relationship of the PFMs and the abdominals is all about power and protection for your female parts. If you over-grip the transversus abdominis, you start to over-activate the other abdominal muscles such as the obliques; this is a big no-no. This is one of the reasons many traditional core programs fail. But my program succeeds because we first aim to correct the diastasis dysfunction and then we create core and pelvic power by strengthening without over-activating the PFMs (which could lead to more spasms, leaking and pain). Also remember that if you are over-gripping you will most likely start to hold your breath which creates an increase in intra-abdominal pressure—another no-no. Any increase in intra-abdominal pressure can lead to organ prolapse, increased leaking and PFM spasms. The New Core is all about conscious awareness, being fully present and not trying too hard to achieve the exercise.

This New Core should be performed by women when they have mastered the reverse Kegel exercise and are on the contract/relax Kegel program. I include this guideline here because I don't want you to experience more pelvic pain and spasms. At the bare minimum, you should close up the diastasis and work on training your transverse abdominal muscles. This is the way to start if you have progressed to the contract/relax Kegel program. Make sure to read and practice the exercises in Chapter 6 that work for you before attempting the New Core for female pelvic power.

Now is the time to reclaim your body and to work within your fitness and symptom levels. First, I will describe what a diastasis recti separation is and how to test yourself for one. Then I will prescribe two corrective exercises to close up the separation and get you back on the road to reclaiming your pelvic power. The New Core Program includes eight levels, which can be found in Table 8.2. Before starting any of the exercises it is important to understand how to keep a neutral spine as most abdominal exercises will require this alignment. Practice neutral spine first and make sure you have it mastered and then embark on your journey to a more powerful core.

I have also included Table 8.3, which details the most common mistakes made while training the abdominal muscles using the New Core for Female Pelvic Power. Familiarize yourself with these common mistakes so that you don't repeat them as you progress in your core program. Once you have the proper foundation and your diastasis recti separation is closed up, you can then start on the New Core training for stronger abdominal muscles and lifelong female pelvic power. Now let's get started.

Specific Considerations for Abdominal Diastasis Recti Separation and the New Core Routine

Diastasis recti abdominis (DRA) is a separation of the rectus abdominis muscle at the linea alba. The outermost abdominal muscles, called the rectus abdominis, form two halves, called right and left recti muscles. These two halves are covered by fibrous connective tissue from other muscles and join at the central seam called the linea alba. Like a zipper, these abdominal muscles can separate due to incorrect biomechanics, pregnancy, with sudden weight gain and obesity. DRA can also result from performing abdominal exercises incorrectly or by suddenly sitting up straight in bed from a horizontal lying down position, called "jackknifing."

DRA has profound effects on the function of the pelvic floor muscles and bladder and bowel function. It is a well-known fact that the PFMs and the abdominals have a synergistic relationship. When DRA is present, it decreases the ability of the PFMs to contract effectively, contributing to urinary, stress and fecal incontinence and sexual dysfunction. DRA leaves the abdominals in a weakened state. When this separation is present in women with pelvic pain, the PFMs cannot function optimally which makes the contract/relax exercises more difficult than they need to be. Make sure to test for DRA as defined in the next section. I would recommend not beginning the core series until your DRA measures two-fingers wide or less. Ideally I like the DRA to measure one-finger width as I find too much dysfunction with the PFMs when the separation is bigger.

It is also important to note that the function and insertion of the other abdominal muscles, called the transversus abdominis and internal/external obliques, are hindered when you have a DRA. This altered state of the abdominals can lead to the formation of trigger points in the abdominal wall. These abdominal trigger points can cause urinary urgency, pelvic pain and refer pain to the vulvar-vaginal area including the bladder. Many times these abdominal trigger points can lead to pain above the pubic bone and can cause the sensation of bladder infections without actually having one. Not only does the DRA need to be corrected, but also all of the abdominal trigger points need to be resolved in order to achieve symptom relief.

Before beginning the New Core program, you must first determine if you have a DRA by performing the test described below. If you find a DRA, perform the corrective exercises in order to close the gap before progressing to the more advanced core program. There are two exercises that you can perform to correct your DRA, one seated and one lying down on your back. If you have very weak abdominal muscles, start with the seated exercise and then incorporate the lying down corrective exercise in one week. It takes time to close up a DRA separation. Closing a DRA requires that you are consistent with the exercises and that you consider the "Tips to Avoid Making the DRA Worse."

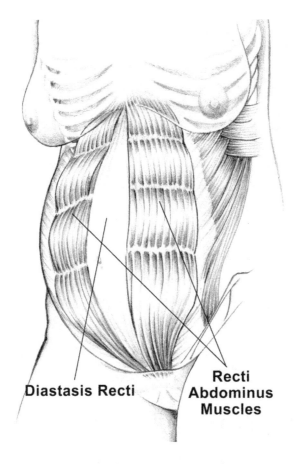

Diastasis Recti   **Recti Abdominus Muscles**

Source for Base Image: Winston Johnson

Tracking DRA Progress

It is important to track your DRA with a chart. It helps you to determine whether you need to increase the number of times you are doing the corrective exercise. I also think it's encouraging to see your progress as you do the hard work.

Table 8.1 DRA Tracking

Use this chart to keep track of your progress as you work to close your DRA.

Date	2 Inches Above	At Umbilicus	2 Inches Below

How to Test for DRA Separation

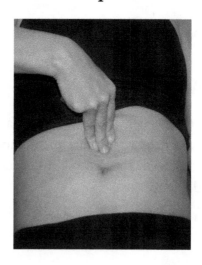

1. Lie on your back with your knees bent.

2. Exhale and slightly lift your head off the floor with your arms reaching forward. Check how many fingers you are able to insert horizontally two inches above the umbilicus, at the umbilicus, and two inches below the umbilicus. Do not engage your abs - it will give you a false positive DRA test. Your DRA will appear smaller than it actually is.

3. DRA of one- to two-fingers separation is considered normal. A three-finger separation requires correction. Corrective exercises are used to close up any separation of the abdominals. The closer the DRA is the less symptomatic you will be. If you still have symptoms at two-finger width, then you need to correct it first. DRA correction in my protocol is driven by symptoms, and for some women, the separation must be closed up to one-finger width. Always test at the same spots as indicated above. If you test at different spots your measurements will be inconsistent.

Tips to Avoid Making the DRA Worse

1. Avoid jackknifing out of bed. Instead, logroll out of bed by engaging your abdominals, turning completely to the side and then use your arms to push yourself to a seated position.

2. Avoid sudden weight gains.

3. Avoid yoga exercises that stretch the abdominals.

4. Avoid coughing or sneezing without first engaging your abdominals.

5. Avoid traditional abdominal exercises such as abdominal crunches, which can make the DRA larger.

6. Avoid exercises at the gym or daily activities that make your belly pop out, also called the diastasis recti bulge.

7. Avoiding leaning forward such as bending from the hips to pick something up from the floor.

8. Avoid pushing and straining with bowel and bladder functions.

9. Avoid abdominal exercises that involve twisting or rotational movements.

10. Avoid standing in poor posture where your back is arched and your belly is sticking out. This includes standing with your knees locked.

Finding Neutral Spine (NS)

Before we start with the corrective exercise for DRA, it is very important that you understand how to maintain and achieve neutral spine. Neutral spine is the natural position of the spine when all the parts of the spine, cervical, thoracic and lumbar, are in excellent alignment. This position is the most favorable when performing the New Female Pelvic Power Core program because it allows your abdominals and PFMs to optimally contract and relax as needed.

Neutral Spine (NS)

WHAT TO DO:

1. Lie on your back with your knees bent and your feet flat on the floor. Make sure your lower extremity is in great alignment. Imagine there is one continuous line from your hips to your knees to your feet. To accomplish this make sure your feet are parallel and not out to the side.

2. Keep your arms at your side and keep the body relaxed.

3. Exhale and use your abdominal muscles to press your lower back into the floor performing a posterior pelvic tilt (PPT). Inhale through your nose into your belly and release the PPT.

4. Exhale and pull your lower spine up and away from the floor creating an anterior pelvic tilt (ANT). Inhale and relax and release the ANT.

5. Most women have their spines either in an anterior pelvic tilt or a posterior pelvic tilt because of muscle imbalances and weakness. Neutral spine is a place in between these two extreme positions. You must practice this until you get a sense of what it means to be in neutral spine for you. Practice this exercise and know how to do it before moving forward.

Corrective DRA Exercises: Seated Splinted Holds

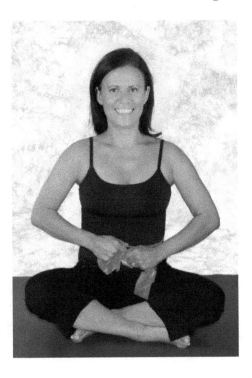

WHAT TO DO:

1. Sit in cross-legged position with correct posture, shoulders over hips or in good posture in a chair.

2. Crisscross your hands over your belly, or use a scarf or Dyna-Band to bring the abdominals together.

3. Inhale through your nose into your belly. Exhale through your mouth to initiate the belly button reaching toward your spine, and up towards the heart, engaging the abdominals while keeping a neutral spine. Hold this position.

4. Simultaneously, pull the sides of your abdominals together with your arms to approximate the recti muscles. Do a gentle PFM contraction while doing the exercise.

5. Breathe naturally and hold for five seconds. Return to start position.

6. Perform 20 times, two to three times a day.

Corrective DRA Exercises: Lying Down Splinted Head Raises

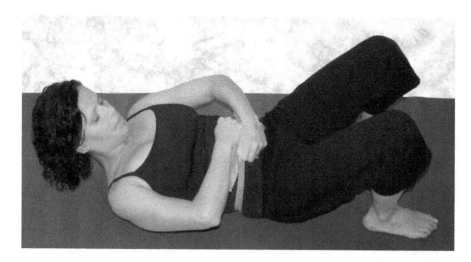

WHAT TO DO:

1. Lie on your back with your knees bent on the floor.

2. Bring your belly button gently to your spine, and draw it up to your heart, while maintaining a NS.

3. Crisscross your hands over your belly, or use a scarf or Dyna-Band to bring the abdominals together while doing Number 2.

4. Exhale very slowly, and raise your head toward your chest just before the diastasis bulge begins. To begin, keep the shoulders in contact with the floor. To maximize the approximation of the recti muscles you can use a large scarf or wrap to bring the muscles together. Do a gentle PFM contraction while doing this exercise.

5. Breathe naturally and hold for five seconds. Return to start position. As you get stronger, you will be able to lift your shoulders off the floor.

6. Perform 20 times, two to three times a day.

Your Diastasis Recti Is Corrected: What Now?

Once you have corrected your diastasis recti and it is within a one to two-finger separation, you are now ready to embark on the more difficult core exercises of the Female Pelvic Power Program. All of the exercises in this amazing program involve a transverse belly hold. You must master this foundational exercise first, before progressing through the rest of the New Core program.

How to Progress in the Abdominal Program

There are several exercises to the New Core program for female pelvic power. It is important not to move to a more difficult exercise before you master the previous level. When you can perform 20 reps, two to three times in great form you have mastered that level and can move to the next level. You can be working at two levels at the same time on different exercises as long as you have mastered the previous level.

THE NEW CORE FOR FEMALE PELVIC POWER

Table 8.2 The New Core for Female Pelvic Power

Corrective DRA Exercises, Seated or Lying Down Level 1
Transverse Belly Holds: Foundational exercise for all other exercises: Level 1
Leg Press: Level 2
Marching: Level 3
Up-Up/Down-Down: Level 4
Toe Taps: Level 5
Bicycles: Level 6
Planks: Level 7
Side Planks: Level 8

Table 8.3 Common Mistakes: What to Avoid in Your Female Pelvic Power Training Program

1. Avoid holding your breath while performing your abdominal exercises. If you hold the breath, you could leak urine, push the organs downward, create PFMs spasms and not activate the core muscles correctly.
2. Do not advance to a more difficult abdominal exercise without first mastering the previous level.
3. Never leak urine. If you leak with your abdominal exercises, then the exercise is too difficult for you. You should return to the previous level and master those exercises without leaking.
4. Do not exacerbate your pelvic pain. There is a thin line between intelligent working out and creating more tension in the abdominal and PFMs. If you experience an increase in pain, you should return to the previous level and master those exercises without pain.
5. Avoid sticking your butt into the air when performing exercises such as plank. If you find that you are sticking out your butt, then you are using too much of your arm and leg power and performing it wrong.
6. Do not flare out your ribs when doing the core program. Instead keep them pulled in toward your spine. If your ribs pop out, then you are not activating the core properly.
7. Avoid sagging the lower back when performing your plank exercises.
8. Do not over-contract your abdominal core muscles. Over-contraction activates the obliques instead of the deeper transversus abdominis muscle. You are over-contracting if you feel a bearing-down sensation in the pelvis or if your lower abdominals "pop out" with contraction. You may also feel increased pelvic pressure if you over activate the abdominal core muscles.
9. Do not forget to co-contract the PFMs with the transverse holds while performing the New Core exercises. True core strength requires activation of both muscle groups through the entire set of exercises. This co-contraction is at about 20 to 30 percent of effort, not 100 percent. Remember: PFM is a low-level contraction.
10. Avoid rounding or arching the lower back while performing the core exercises. Keep your spine in neutral while performing all the exercises.

Transverse Belly Holds

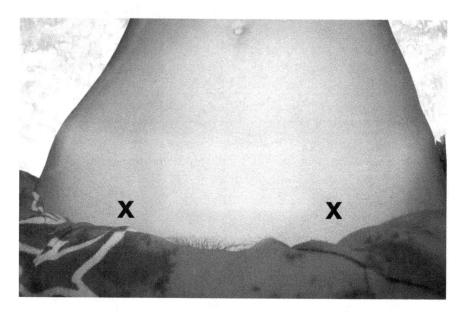

WHAT TO DO:

1. This exercise may be done sitting, supine, standing, or on all fours. Keep a neutral spine as you inhale. Then, as you exhale, draw your belly button gently inward and up towards your heart. As you engage the Transverse Belly Hold, try to imagine that you are squeezing into an old pair of jeans that don't fit, and maintain a neutral spine.

2. Additional cues that work well to activate and train the transverse muscle are:

    a. Imagine that you are doing a Kegel that moves all the way up to the lower part of your abdominals and travels to your heart.

    b. Imagine that there is a guy wire from the right anterior hip bone to the left and imagine the guy wire becoming slack as you bring the two hip bones together.

3. Once you establish the above movement, hold for five seconds and repeat ten times. Do one to three sets per day. Use the different cues to help you. Although this exercise looks easy it is extremely difficult to train and isolate the transverse muscle. This exercise is the building block for all the exercises that follow so take your time and practice it.

WHAT TO WATCH OUT FOR:

1. Holding the breath, which can increase leaking or pelvic pain.

2. Over-contracting the abdominals, which engages the more superficial abdominals, such as the rectus abdominis and external obliques.

3. Increased abdominal pain or trigger points in the abdominals and/or an increase in your symptoms.

Leg Press

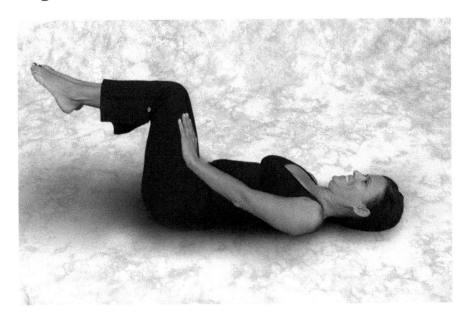

WHAT TO DO:

1. Lie flat on the floor with your lower back in NS and rest your arms on the side. Engage your transversus abdominis and your PFMs. Keep this engagement at 20 to 30 percent of effort.

2. Hug your knees into your chest, then release your knees slightly away from you until they form a 90 degree angle.

3. Bring your outstretched hand or hands to your thighs and gently push your hands into your thighs making sure your legs don't move. Continue this pressing into your thighs for five seconds and then rest. Repeat ten times or as tolerated.

4. You may also try this in a seated position with your feet flat on the floor. This is a great exercise to do at work.

WHAT TO WATCH OUT FOR:

1. Moving the legs and pressing too hard. This exercise is a sustained hold with no movement.

2. Holding the breath. Breathe naturally as you hold the resistance against your thighs.

3. Allowing the rectus abdominis to "pop out" during the exercise. If your belly bulges or your back comes off the floor, then you have likely lost your transverse belly hold and the NS.

Marching

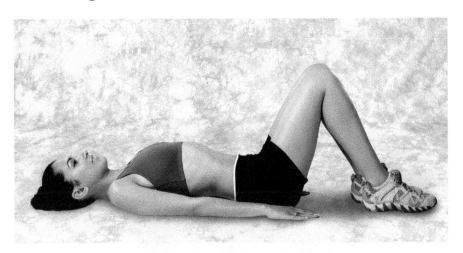

WHAT TO DO:

1. Lie flat on the floor with a NS and rest your arms on the side. Engage your transversus abdominis and your PFMs. Keep this engagement at 20 to 30 percent of effort.

2. Slowly raise the right leg one to three inches from the floor. Keep trunk rigid. Hold three seconds. Lower the right leg and then slowly raise the left leg one to three inches from the floor. Keep trunk rigid. Hold for three seconds.

3. Repeat ten times on each leg.

4. Remember to keep the hips still and stable while performing this exercise. Do not move back and forth as you switch legs.

WHAT TO WATCH OUT FOR:

1. Holding the breath, which can increase leaking or pelvic pain.

2. Over-contracting, which engages the more superficial abdominals, such as the rectus abdominis and external obliques.

3. Moving the pelvis and trunk and lifting the legs too high off the floor.

Up-Up/Down-Down

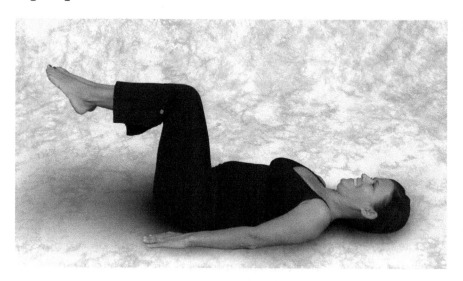

WHAT TO DO:

1. Lie flat on the floor with a NS and rest your arms on the side. Engage your transversus abdominis and your PFMs. Keep this engagement at 20 to 30 percent of effort.

2. Hug your knees into your chest, then release your knees slightly away from you until they form a 90 degree angle.

3. Holding the trunk stable and maintaining a transverse belly hold, release the right knee slightly away from you, then release the left to meet the right. This is the "down-down" position.

4. Then draw the right knee back up to 90 degrees followed by the left. This is the "up-up" position.

5. Continue in this down-down, up-up movement pattern for 20 reps. Maintain NS throughout the exercise. Repeat eight to ten times with the goal of reaching 20 reps.

WHAT TO WATCH OUT FOR:

1. Holding the breath, which can increase leaking or pelvic pain.

2. Over-contracting, which engages the more superficial abdominals, such as the rectus abdominis and external obliques.

3. The down-down position is the hardest position. Avoid arching your back, as this can cause a strain or injury to the lower back.

Toe Taps

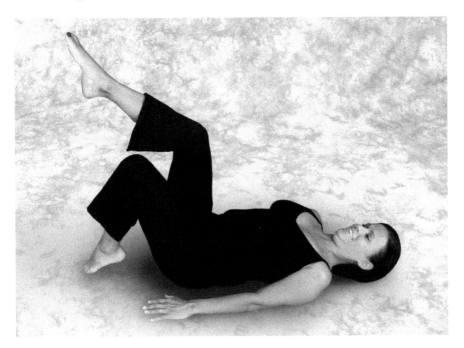

WHAT TO DO:

1. Lie flat on the floor with a NS and rest your arms on the side. Engage your transverse abdominal muscles and your PFMs. Keep this engagement at 20 to 30 percent of effort.

2. Start by hugging your knees into your chest, then release your knees slightly away from you until they form a 90 degree angle.

3. Slowly lower right leg toward the floor (keep your knees bent to tap your toes to the floor). Once you tap the right toe, raise your leg back up to the start position. Then lower your left leg until the toe touches the floor or mat. Once you tap the left toe, raise your leg back up to the start position.

4. Continue in this pattern of right toe touch, back to start position and then left toe touch for 20 reps. Repeat for two to three sets or as tolerated.

WHAT TO WATCH OUT FOR:

1. Holding the breath, which can increase leaking, pelvic pressure or pelvic pain.

2. Performing the toe taps too quickly, which will hinder the effectiveness of this exercise. Focus on performing the exercise correctly, with a transverse belly hold and minimal rocking of the pelvis.

3. Avoid arching your lower back, as this can cause a strain or injury to the lower back.

4. Moving the pelvis and hips too much and doing the exercise too quickly.

Bicycles

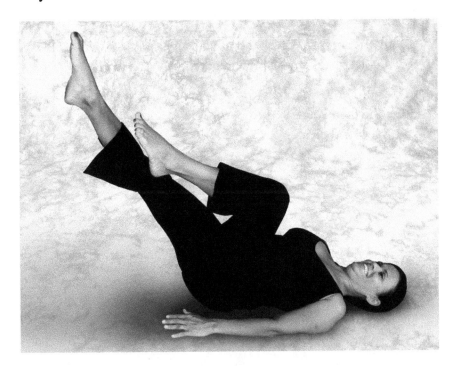

WHAT TO DO:

1. Lie flat on the floor with a NS and rest your arms on the side. Engage your transversus abdominis and your PFMs. Keep this engagement at 20 to 30 percent of effort.

2. Bring your knees up to about a 90 degree angle and slowly go through a bicycle pedal motion as pictured. This should be a smooth and fluid motion as if you are riding a bicycle. Keep the legs high. The lower your legs are the more difficult this exercise becomes. It is best to start with a high bicycle and then lower the legs when you are super strong.

3. Perform the exercise in a slow, controlled motion. Repeat 10 to 20 times on each side.

WHAT TO WATCH OUT FOR:

1. Performing the exercise too quickly and losing the form and control.

2. Avoid arching your low back, as this can cause a strain or injury to the lower back muscles, which help stabilize the core.

3. Performing the bicycle with the legs too low, which is very difficult when you are not ready to do so. Be careful not to injure your back and create spasms in the PFMs.

Planks

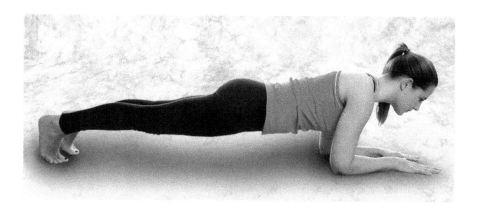

WHAT TO DO:

1. Get into push-up position on the floor. Engage your transverse abdominis and your PFMs. Now bend your elbows 90 degrees and rest your weight on your forearms. Your elbows should be directly beneath your shoulders, and your body should form a straight line from your head to your feet.

2. Hold the plank position for ten seconds or as tolerated. The goal here would be 60-second holds. Repeat five to ten times. If this exercise is too difficult make it easier by placing your knees on the floor. Remember to lift the feet off the floor for this easier version. (Note: This version of the exercise is not shown in the photograph.)

WHAT TO WATCH OUT FOR:

1. Keep your spine straight and do not stick your butt into the air.

2. Avoid arching your low back, as this can cause a strain or injury to the lower back. Keep your spine in neutral.

Side Planks

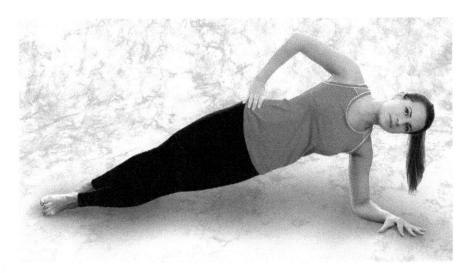

WHAT TO DO:

1. Lie on your side on the mat. Place your forearm on the mat, directly under and perpendicular to your body. Place your upper leg directly on top of your lower leg and straighten your knees and hips. Engage your transverse abdominis and your PFMs.

2. Raise your body upward by straightening the waist, so that your body is stable and rigid. Hold position. Repeat with opposite side.

3. Hold the side plank position for ten seconds or as tolerated. Repeat five to ten times.

WHAT TO WATCH OUT FOR:

1. Keep position straight and do not sag in the middle of the body.

2. Breathe naturally.

3. Make sure the DRA is closed. Side planks can open the DRA so always test your DRA to make sure you haven't reopened it with this exercise.

Now that our foundation is almost set, let's build upon this and examine our bladders in more detail. Chapter 4 discusses the bladder but in the next chapter I give you additional tools that, when incorporated into your healing program, will bring great results. Make sure to go back and re-read Chapter 4 before progressing to Chapter 9. Together both chapters will teach you how to tame and control your bladder and your symptoms. So read on...

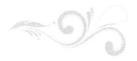

You have come this far, but I have more to teach you.

The Truth About Training Your Abdominal Muscles

…to go deeper ONLINE, visit
http://www.FemalePelvicAlchemy.com/chapter8

I've got something super cool waiting for you here:
A special training video that will help you to understand
how to get really powerful, beautiful and toned
abdominals while improving your sexual power and function.
This is truly a gift. Don't miss out….

CHAPTER 9

Energy Medicine That Awakens Your Feminine Sexuality

Keeping the pelvic floor healthy supple, flexible and clear can be achieved with massage and energy exercises that target the chakra system. The chakra circulate energy in the body and this energy is call *chi*. Chi is within us and within all our organs. It's the universal energy/life source. When the energies are circulating, we feel connected and healthy. Many women have too much chi, too little chi, or blocked chi, creating an imbalance that leads to sexual dysfunction, pain, lack of pleasure or pelvic congestion. The goal is to have the right amount of chi so that we have great pleasure and great orgasms, while feeling connected to ourselves and the world around us.

The women that I treat sometimes tell me that they feel as if something is out of alignment and that things just don't feel right in their vaginas or in their bodies. When the energy is out of balance or when the chakras are closed, we feel closed off and disconnected. There are exercises that open the chakra system and balance our chi energy so we feel more in sync with our female power. The more open our chakras are the healthier and more connected we feel.

There are 7 major chakras and we will be focusing on them with the exercises and massages in this chapter. Also note that there are 21 minor chakras, which are equally important, but beyond the scope of this book. The locations of the seven major chakras are seen in the photograph below. They are in straight row alignment; chakra one starts at the bottom and they ascend the body until they reach the crown. Each major chakra in the front is paired off with a back chakra at the same location.

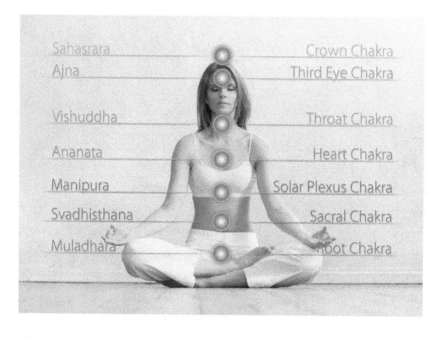

Sahasrara — Crown Chakra
Ajna — Third Eye Chakra
Vishuddha — Throat Chakra
Ananata — Heart Chakra
Manipura — Solar Plexus Chakra
Svadhisthana — Sacral Chakra
Muladhara — Root Chakra

The pelvic floor muscles live in the first chakra, and if those muscles are out of balance, chances are you will feel out of sorts also. There are 7 major chakras and 21 minor chakras, but I focus primarily on the first chakra since this is the building block of all our energetic bodies.

Each chakra has a specific location, color, organ, gland and one of the five senses associated with it. (Refer to Table 9.1 for additional information on chakra associations.) Chakras are also associated with psychological function and the energy fields. As you can see this system is a complex network and can take a lifetime to learn. If you are interested in exploring the energy fields and the complete chakra system further, I encourage you to do additional independent research on the topic.

Table 9.1 Location and Color of the Seven Chakras

Chakra Number	Location	Color
1	Pelvic floor muscles	Red
2	Sacrum	Orange
3	Solar plexus-under the breast bone but above the navel	Yellow
4	Heart-center of chest	Green
5	Throat	Blue
6	Third eye-area between the brows	Indigo
7	Crown-top of head	Violet

As a Reiki practitioner I frequently work with patients to clear their blocked chakras. I incorporate chakra opening exercises into their programs and I will show you the exercises that have brought many of my patients long-term healing and connectedness. First, we'll briefly review the chakra system.

The first chakra is called the base chakra and is located within the pelvic floor. This is the chakra that is responsible for how safe you feel in the world. Women with sexual trauma and/or injuries to the first chakra do not feel safe and can sometimes close off the opening to their vaginas. This is not a conscious act but a byproduct of their experiences. I treat a lot of sexual pain and pelvic floor muscle hypertonicity (non-relaxing PFMs), and I have found a correlation between a closed-off first chakra and sexual trauma.

The second chakra is located at the level of the sacrum and houses the reproductive organs and sexual activity. Located at the solar plexus, the third chakra houses our emotions such as self-worth, self-esteem and our past traumas. The fourth chakra, the heart chakra, is located in the center of the chest and helps us to connect our divine selves to our physical selves. Typically, women who have had bad relationships or who have experienced nasty divorces have a problem with this chakra. I also find this chakra can be closed off due to issues with parents. This is the heart, so basically all matters of the heart—bad or good—can affect this chakra. It is important to remain open in the heart chakra because love is what rules the world and self-love is the most important love of all.

The fifth or throat chakra can become affected when we swallow our words and cannot speak our truths. Many times I find that women will not speak out to their partners about their sexual preferences. They might even be faking orgasms to please their partners. When we are connected to our true selves and know our power, we can more easily express what we feel. The chakra throat exercise will connect you to your inner power and you will find that you will more easily express feelings that you may have been reluctant to reveal. When we express our inner truths we feel better about ourselves and that impacts our relationships as well.

The sixth chakra is located at our third eye and is connected to our womanly senses—our deep intuition. How many times have you told yourself: "I wish I listened to my gut"? When this chakra is open we can experience and trust the magic of our inner voices and connect to what our bodies, spirit and mind are telling us. The seventh or crown chakra is how we connect to the divine or to our "goddess" or "goddess-self." When this chakra is closed off we feel disconnected, depressed and don't trust our paths. Maybe we don't trust the universe anymore or maybe we are angry at the goddess. Maybe we have faulty thinking. Maybe we are always thinking the worst could happen or "I'll never get better." (Don't skip the exercise for the crown chakra: it's as important as all the others.)

When your chakras are well nourished and open, you feel like you can fly and you bounce back much easier from difficulty and disease. You feel a sense of deep connection to everything around you and to your goddess self. That's my goal: for you to feel this beautiful energy flowing through you so that you are healthy not only in the pelvic area but throughout your body.

Goddess Bodywork

In addition to specific chakra exercises, there are some simple exercises that can help create flexibility and suppleness in the pelvic floor muscles, thereby creating more balance. I've named this series of integrative exercises targeted to move female chi **"Goddess Bodywork"** because you should think of yourself as a goddess worthy of love. The sexual alchemical exercises that comprise Goddess Bodywork help build chi and balance the chakras with massages and stretching. Breath Work and meditation, key components of the series, enable you to harvest and balance energy. Pelvic and sexual healing exercises as well as sound healing for the vulva round out the series.

You will find that with Goddess Bodywork you will recapture your sexual energy and enhance balance, flexibility and suppleness within the pelvic floor muscles. The series also serves as excellent preparation for the Alchemical Kegels. The end result will be overall better bladder, bowel and sexual function. You can do the entire Goddess Bodywork series or opt to just do parts of it. Of course, these exercises are vigorous and can produce soreness. Listen to your body and avoid going into pain.

The chart below lists all the exercises and techniques that make up the Goddess Bodywork series; we will explore each in great detail. If you are new to this type of exercising start with one set of 10 three times a week with one day of rest in-between sessions. Once you have mastered the exercises then you can progress to the more advanced version of daily work and increase your sets from 1 to 3.

Table 9.2 The Goddess Bodywork Series

Abdominal Rolling: Large Abdominal Clockwise Circles
Psoas Release
Upper Thigh and Inner Thigh Clockwise Circles
External Vulvar Massage Clockwise
Labia Rolling
Labia Stretching
Legs Up the Wall Toes In
Legs Up the Wall Toes Out
Connective Tissue Massage
Seated Sacral Rolling
Lumbar Massage
Meditation
Tension Release Breathing
Alchemical Breathing or Goddess Meditation
Rock Around the Clock
Chakra Opening Exercises 1 to 7
Inner Smile Energy Exercise
Sound Healing for the Vulva: Techniques 1 to 6

Abdominal Rolling: Large Abdominal Clockwise Circles

The PFMs are influenced by the fascia of the abdominal muscles. When the PFMs are painful, in spasms, and lack mobility, the abdominal muscle can sometimes respond by becoming tight, painful and developing trigger points. When abdominal massage and rolling are incorporated into treatment, patients are better able to tolerate the intravaginal stretches and massage more easily. Many of my patients tell me that after the abdominal massage they can insert their dilator or finger into their vaginas with more ease and less pain. The abdominal muscles may also have trigger points in them, and you will discover yours as you massage and explore the abdominals.

To facilitate abdominal rolling, place a heating pad or hot water bottle on your tummy for ten minutes before you start rolling. Use low heat: Avoid high heat because you could burn yourself. You can roll the abdominal muscles with or without an oil. First, try rolling without an oil; if that is too painful then think about using aromatherapy and choose an oil that helps you to relax and glide over the abdominal muscle with ease and little or no pain. Try *Young Living Oils* to help release pain, spasms and help with digestion; I most frequently use lavender and peppermint for the abdominals.

Precaution for Abdominal Rolling:

Your physician will provide the guidelines, but generally you must wait six weeks after abdominal surgery before starting these techniques. (Also check with your doctor if you are recovering from another type of surgery.) This is when the abdominal scar is almost fully healed. Your doctor may give you permission to start earlier, but you should only begin abdominal rolling/massage any earlier than six weeks after abdominal or laparoscopic surgery with medical clearance.

Also check with your MD regarding time frames for Cesarean or myomectomy surgeries.

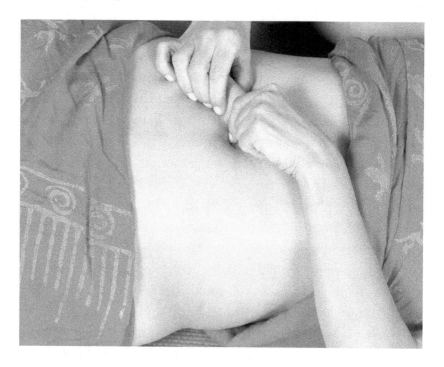

WHAT TO DO:

1. Get pleasant aromatherapy oil with a scent that helps you to relax as you work with your abdominal rolling. Lavender oil is a lovely scent and helps reduce bladder symptoms. I use *Young Living Oils.* You can order these at *www.youngliving.com/en_US/* and use my number #1422496 when ordering. Make sure to obtain medical clearance from your MD before using any aromatherapy oils.

2. Cup your abdominal muscles by placing index fingers near each other so they are gently touching and place your thumbs superior to the other fingers as in the photo above. Stay superficial on your abdominal muscle and avoid grabbing the muscles too deeply.

3. Gently glide your fingers toward your thumbs repeating 10 to 20 times and change your hand placement. For simplicity's sake, I have divided the abdominal muscles into an upper part and lower part. Roll the lower part first, focusing on upward motions. Make sure to cover all the lower abdominal muscles and then switch to rolling the upper abdominal muscles in a downward motion.

4. Remember to pay attention to trigger points. If you come across a very painful trigger point – and sometimes these painful spots can refer pain elsewhere in the pelvis – hold the spot for 90 seconds until the pain subsides. Repeat the 90-second holds until you have either eliminated the trigger point or reduced the pain by 50 percent.

5. Finish your abdominal rolling by gently massaging your entire abdominal region with clockwise circles.

6. Try to roll your abdominals 5 to 15 minutes on a daily basis and perform at least 20 clockwise circles to end your massage.

Psoas Release

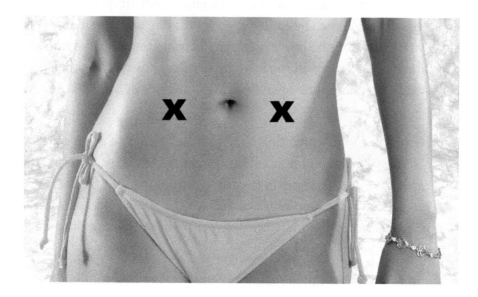

Your body has two very deep muscles on either side of the lower abdomen called the psoas muscles. These muscles attach from the lower spine to the hip bones, and help flex the hips. The psoas muscles are frequently very painful, in spasm, and irritated in women suffering from pelvic pain. The psoas release technique increases blood flow to the pelvis and is highly effective in reducing pain and normalizing PFMs tension and function. It is also great for women who have low back pain.

To find the psoas muscles do the following:

1. Lie on your back with your legs straight out.

2. Go about two to three inches to the right side of your belly button. Place your fingertips into the area, slowly allowing them to sink into your abdomen and being careful to avoid any feelings of an artery pulse.

3. Lift your right leg straight up and you will feel the psoas pop into your hand. It may take a little practice to get this but keep trying. Once you know where the psoas muscle is, place your fingertips in that spot and slowly press downward into the psoas for 60 to 90 seconds. If you feel any tingling, numbness, or tremendous increase in pain, get off the area and try to relocate the psoas muscle. Switch sides and do the left psoas muscle release.

4. CAUTION HERE: Do not press into an area that has a pulse. If you feel a pulse, move to a different area and locate the muscle at another place.

Upper Thigh and Inner Thigh Clockwise Circles

1. Lie on the floor and bend knees, with feet hip-width apart.

2. Place palms on thighs and imagine white healing loving light coming out of the middle of your palm as you massage your thighs in clockwise circles. Complete three sets of 20 circles.

External Vulvar Massage Clockwise

Place palms on vulva and imagine white healing loving light coming out of the middle of your palm as you massage your vulva in clockwise circles. Complete three sets of 20 circles and repeat three times.

Labia Rolling

Pinch the right labia majora between the thumb and the forefinger. Roll the tissue gently between the fingers until you reach the bottom. You can roll the labia tissue in either an upward or downward direction; choose the direction that is least painful for you. Repeat 2 to 3 times and then switch sides. Be very gentle and soft when working on this delicate structure.

Labia Stretching

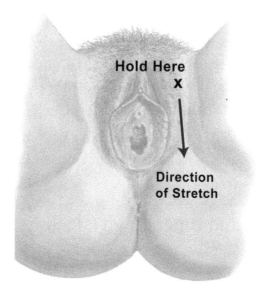

Source: Netter Images.

Anchor your finger on the top of the right labia majora near the clitoris. Place the thumb of the opposite hand at the bottom of the same labia and stretch downward. Hold for 30 seconds to 1 minute, repeating 2 to 3 times and then switch to the other labia.

Legs Up the Wall Toes In

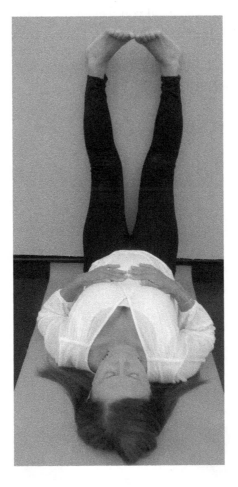

1. Lie face up near a wall with your buttocks as close to the wall as possible, and your legs up the wall.

2. Keep your hips and lower back flat on the floor. Place a small pillow under pelvis for comfort.

3. Keep your body relaxed while you move both feet apart from each other.

4.   Point your toes inward.

5.   Only open your legs until you feel a mild to medium stretch in your inner thigh muscles. Hold for one complete breath cycle.

6.   CAUTION HERE: this exercise should not be performed during the menstrual cycle.

Legs Up the Wall Toes Out

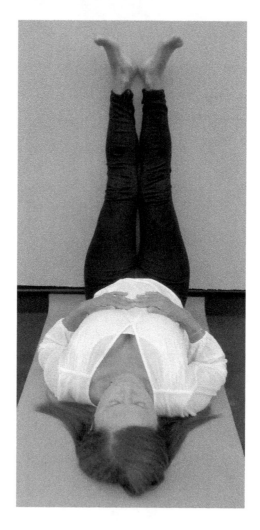

Follow the instructions for **Legs Up the Wall Toes In,** but modify the exercise. Point your toes outward and hold for one breath cycle. CAUTION HERE: this exercise should not be performed during the menstrual cycle.

Connective Tissue Massage

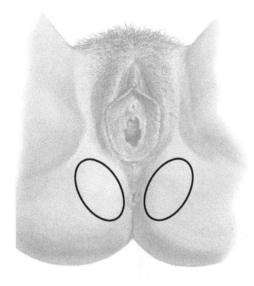

The circles indicate where the ischioanal rolling should be performed.
Source: Netter Images.

1. The ischioanal fossa has several borders and the treatment of this area with rolling and massaging cannot be overstated or overlooked.

2. Locate the ischioanal fossa between the sit bone and the anal rim; palpate the soft tissue cavity.

3. Place your fingertips in the lower part of the fossa and the thumbs on the upper part. The idea is to roll the skin of the fossa toward the thumbs. Roll this area up to five minutes. Focus on the most painful side first.

4. You can do this exercise by gripping the fossa underneath the butt check and rolling it upward toward the sit bone.

Sacral Rolling

This technique opens up the nerves to the pelvis and brings profound pain relief while restoring neurological, connective tissue and bony functions. This is the area from where the pudendal nerve arises and we want to keep it free of restrictions. The sacrum houses many of the nerve roots that innervate the abdominal organs, PFMs and hip muscles. It is critical to keep the tissues in this area free and supple. Sacral rolling is a great tool for this.

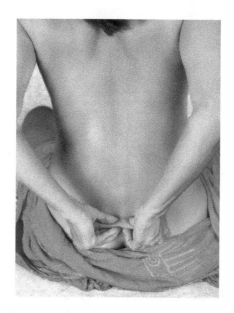

1. Cup the skin in your sacral area and roll it in the same manner that you would roll your abdominals. See the photo for hand placement.

2. Roll the sacrum upward for two to five minutes on a daily basis. In the beginning, sacral rolling might be painful, but over time it will become less painful.

3. The goal is to be pain-free when doing the sacral rolling.

Lumbar Massage

Many of the women I treat with pelvic pain also suffer from lower back pain. These two conditions go hand-in-hand. Massaging the lower back is important to help release tension and trigger points in this region.

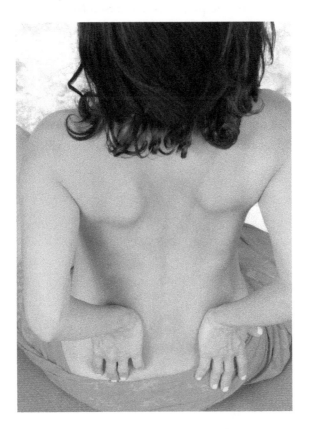

1. Learn to massage yourself in different positions and use firm pressure, avoiding excessive pain.

2. Massage down the lower back muscles using long downward strokes. You can use your knuckles or hands. Make sure to cover the entire lower back area.

3. Using your right hand, massage your right lower back muscles for five to ten minutes. Then switch sides massaging your left lower back muscles with your left hand.

4. For painful trigger points found in any of the back muscles, apply sustained pressure over the painful area for 90 seconds. Repeat as necessary until the pain has decreased by at least 50 percent or the pain is totally eliminated.

5. A great addition to the low back rolling is to massage your low back outward from the spine along the line of your hip bone using your knuckles. This can be very painful at first, but continue to do this massage until the pain has diminished by 50 percent or more. The goal here is to be pain-free.

Meditation

Meditations and mantras empower pelvic pain sufferers to manage stress and overcome negative thinking. A mantra is a repeated word, syllable, phrase, or sound that can help you relax during times of stress. Saying a mantra during meditation or at various times throughout the day will help quiet your mind and bring inner peace to you.

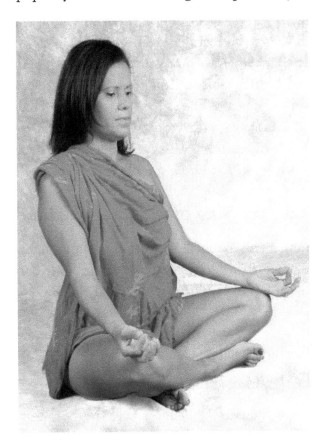

1. Sit or lie down, usually with eyes closed. Focus on deep diaphragmatic breathing for 5 to 10 breaths as you slow down your mind.

2. Begin repeating your mantra with conviction, allowing it to permeate your being.

3. After 3 to 5 minutes, resume diaphragmatic breathing. Repeat the mantra or try a different one.

Tension Release Breathing

In your mind's eye, send your in-breath or inhalation to the part of your muscles where you feel the most tension or pain. Imagine that you are collecting the tension in your muscles with your in-breath. With your out-breath, exhale all the tension out of the muscles. You will learn to relax and ease the tension in your muscles much easier by performing the stretches with proper breathing techniques. Patients who use this type of breathing with their stretching are able to control their pain better, especially during muscle flare-ups.

Alchemical Breathing or Goddess Meditation

This is a centering and connecting breath that put us in touch with our inner goddess and creates long-lasting healing. In my opinion, this is one of the most powerful breaths in the world.

1. Sit in a comfortable position in good posture.

2. Place your right hand on center of chest.

3. Place your left hand at the navel at mid belly.

4. Breathe in and out of the belly, 2nd chakra/the uterus.

5. Breathe in and out of the belly, 4th chakra/the heart.

6. Breathe in and out of the belly, 3rd chakra/the third eye. Continue this breathing cycle for 5 minutes.

Warm Up: Pelvic Clock Circles for Pelvic Healing

If there is one exercise that heals the pelvic floor while simultaneously connecting and opening up the first and second chakras, it is pelvic clock circles. This exercise is the precursor to the chakra opening exercises and for best results you should master the pelvic clocks before moving onto chakra opening exercises. The pelvic clocks can be done on a daily basis for up to one week before moving on to the more advanced chakra opening exercises.

Rock Around the Clock

Imagine a big clock lying on your belly and imagine making pelvic circles around the clock. Now lie on your back with your knees bent and feet on floor. Avoid moving the knees in and out as you do your pelvic clock circles. Stay as pure to the motion as possible.

Imagine that:

- 12 o'clock is located by your clitoris/pubic bone.
  When you move your pelvis to 12 o'clock your tailbone is pointing upward and your lower back is flat on the floor.

- 6 o'clock is located by your anus/coccyx.
  When you move your pelvis to 6 o'clock your tailbone moves back and your lower back is arched.

- 3 o'clock is located by the left side of your body.
  When you move your pelvis to 3 o'clock left pelvis moves toward the floor and right hip lifts up.

- 9 o'clock is located by the right side of your body.
  When you move your pelvis to 9 o'clock right pelvis moves toward the floor and left hip lifts.

Basic Movement:

You are moving in a circular motion in either a clockwise or counterclockwise direction. These circles are easier to do when they are small and more difficult to do when they are larger. You can also do imaginary pelvic circles in your mind to create a mind/body connection.

Breathing:

Now incorporate the breath with the pelvic clock movement to increase mind/body awareness and oxygenation.

Beginner: Gentle normal breathing with clock circles.

Advanced Breathing Work with Kegel and Reverse Kegel: Inhale as you go to the 6 o'clock position and incorporate a reverse Kegel to promote flexibility. Exhale as you go to the 6 o'clock position and perform a Kegel to promote power and strength.

Advanced Breathing Work: Exhale at the upper part of the clock (above the navel at 3, 12, 9 o'clock) positions and inhale at the lower part of clock (below the navel 3, 6, 9 o'clock) positions.

SUMMARY: Pelvic Clock Muscle Healing

Repeat_____/ _____ minutes per day.

Bring Your Goddess Back Home with Chakra Healing

The chakra opening exercises that follow are designed to keep you open while remaining grounded. These exercises help you to remain healthy and unblocked. When chakras are closed, we feel disconnected and out of sorts and blocked energies may even make us ill. Conversely, when our chakras are healthy and open, we are in our groove and in a state of good health. As a Reiki practitioner, I believe all illness starts in the energetic body and then manifests in our physical bodies. With the program that I have outlined here, you will be able to stay healthy and open, and prevent illness, stress and anxiety. When working with the energy body we must listen carefully to what our bodies are telling us. We cannot rush this process. With consistent practice, you will become more and more connected and more and more open.

There are seven chakra exercises, each designed to open a specific chakra. They are quite physical and must be practiced slowly and mindfully. Never push past your discomfort and always remember to rest at the end of the exercises. When resting, imagine that all the chakras are open and working properly. Sometimes you may want to focus more on one chakra than another and that's okay. If possible do the entire chakra routine as a whole. When you perform the exercise series in its entirety you will feel supercharged and ready to take on the world. Sometimes if there are blocks in the chakras you may experience an emotional release which is a good thing. It is important to take note of your feelings and to acknowledge them. No true goddess suppresses her emotions. Live them fully and express them fully but release them. There is no point in holding on to anger and fear. The exercises can be performed on a daily basis or every other day depending on how you feel.

Chakra Opening Exercises[1]
Chakra One: "Be Your Heroine" Exercise

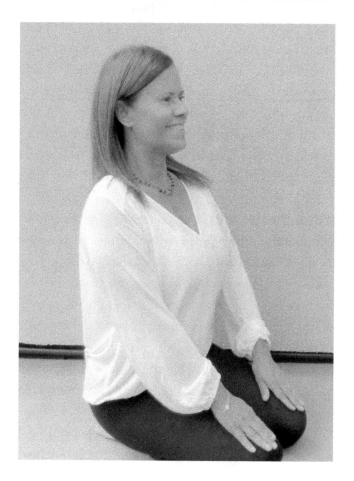

1. Sit back on your heals with your toes turned under and place your outstretched hands on your thighs.

2. Thrust your pelvis back and forth. As you thrust back exhale and allow your spine to flex as long as there's no pain. Repeat 10 times.

---

1   These Chakra Opening Exercises have been adapted from Barbara Brennan's books, *Hands of Light: A Guide to Healing Through the Human Energy Field* and *Light Emerging: The Journey of Personal Healing*. See Bibliography.

Modification:

1. Stand with feet slightly wider than hip-width apart and turn the toes outward so you are in a plié stance. Make sure your knees are not stressed or hurting. Adjust your turn out as needed.

2. Thrust the hips forward and back in a swinging motion. Repeat 10 times.

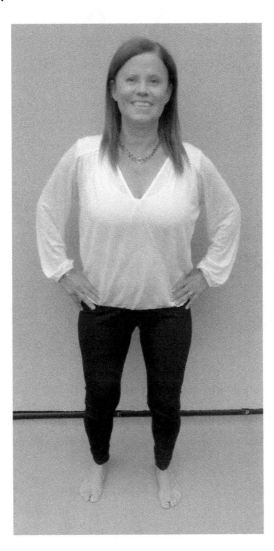

Chakra Two: "The Creative" Exercise

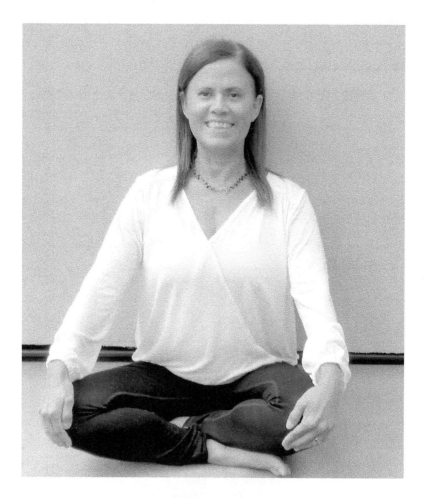

1. Sit pretzel style and grab your ankles with both hands.

2. Thrust your pelvis back and forth. As you thrust back exhale and allow your spine to flex as long as there's no pain. Repeat 10 times.

Modification:

1. Stand with feet shoulder-width apart and feet pointing straight ahead. Make sure your knees are not stressed or hurting.

2. Thrust the hips forward and back in a swinging motion. Repeat 10 times.

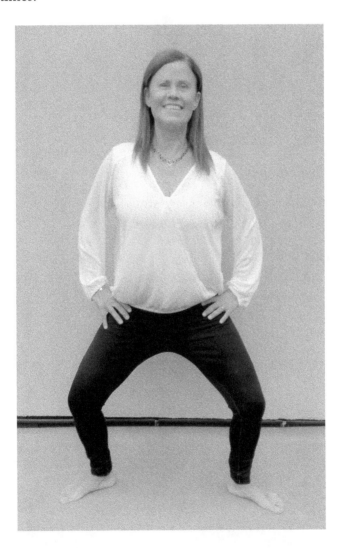

Chakra Three: "Let the Sunshine In" Exercise

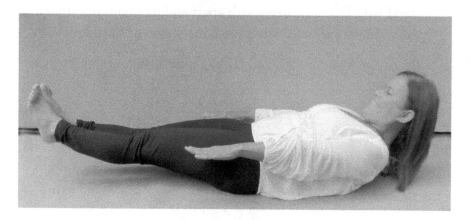

Precaution: You should train your core before doing this chakra exercise and you should have no Diastasis Recti separation.

1. Lie on your back with your legs straight and together and lift them 6 inches off the floor.

2. Lift your head, neck and shoulder about 4 to 6 inches off the floor and breathe in and out of your nose 30 times. To stretch out your back bring your knees to chest.

Modification:

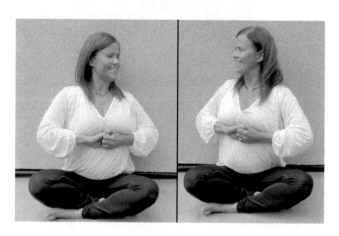

1. Sit pretzel style and place your hands above your navel but below your breast bone and rotate your spine to the left and to the right.

2. As you rotate right exhale and as you rotate left inhale. Repeat 10 times.

Chakra Four: "Heart Connector" Exercise

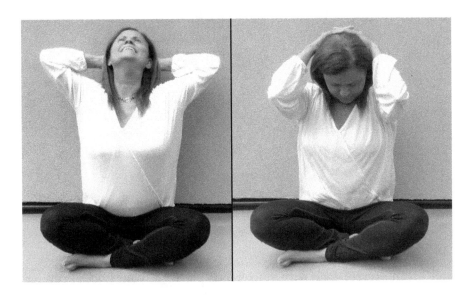

1. Sit in pretzel style with your hands behind your head. Inhale, arch your back and lift your chest.

2. Exhale fold over and flex your upper back. Imagine that you are showing off a beautiful necklace as you arch your upper back.

Modification:

1. Perform the above exercise, sitting in a chair in good posture.

Chakra Five: "Speak the Truth" Exercise

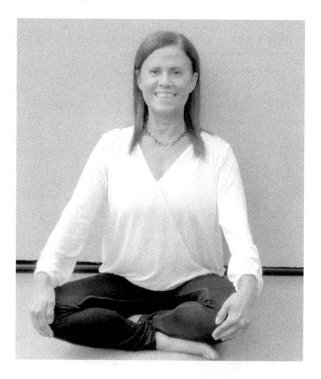

1. Sit in pretzel style with your hands placed at your knees keeping the elbows straight.

2. Look up and open the throat and look down and bring your chin to your chest if you can. Be careful not to aggravate neck pain or cervical herniations.

3. If you have a cervical herniation you will do a chin tuck instead by bringing your chin straight back to your cervical spine. Hold the chin tuck for 3 to 5 seconds and repeat 5 to 10 times or as tolerated.

Chakra Six: "The Ever Seeing" Exercise

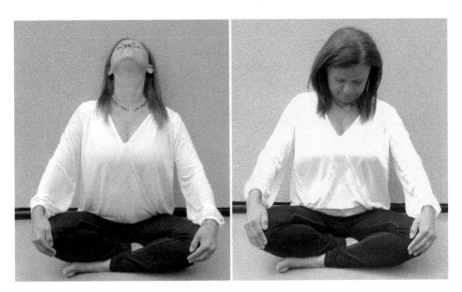

1. Sit in good posture with head in neutral and look straight ahead. Do not move your head just your eyeballs. You will use your eyes here.

2. Look up and then down.

3. Look right and then left.

4. Look up to the right and then down to the left.

5. Look up to the left and then down to the right.

6. This is one full cycle; do 5 to 10 cycles.

Chakra Seven: "Long Live the Queen" Exercise

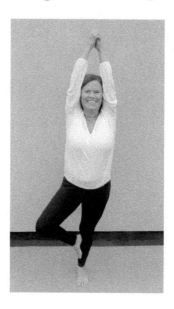

1. This pose helps to ground and open the crown chakra.

2. Stand with feet hip-width apart and keep your back straight and tall.

3. Stare at a focal point in front of you to help you with your balance.

4. Breathe in and lift the right leg and place the sole of your right foot on the left leg upper inner thigh. If this is too difficult you can modify by placing the foot on the calf.

5. Breathe in and raise the arms up, joining the hands with index fingers pointed upward. Elbows should be straight and arms very activated.

6. Hold for 10 to 30 seconds repeat on the other side.

Once your chakras are aligned, open and unblocked you can go about your day. I typically do these exercises before the start of my day so I am clear and focused. Other times I need to rest for a few minutes in order to harvest and integrate. In the beginning you may have to rest, but as you get accustomed to these exercises you can go about your business. My two favorites are Long Legs and Butterfly Legs.

Long Legs

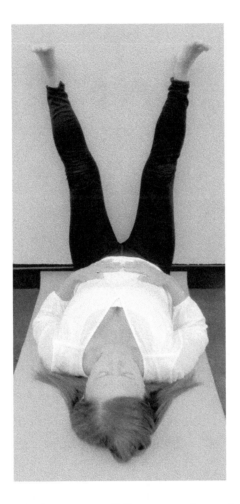

1. Lie on your back close to a wall. Bring your buttocks as close to the wall as possible. Swings your legs up so they are resting on the wall. Your feet are parallel to each other with heels resting on the wall.

2. Place your hands on your belly or place your right hand on your heart and your left hand below your navel and breathe deeply into your belly. You can listen to music or do the Humming exercise that I cover next.

Butterfly Legs

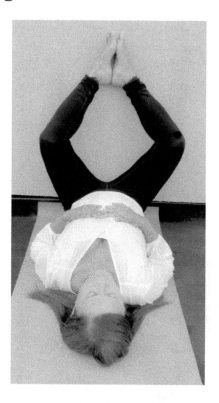

1. Lie on your back close to a wall. Bring your buttocks as close to the wall as possible. Swings your legs up so they are resting on the wall.

2. Bend your legs until the soles of your feet are touching. In this position meditate, hum, tone or just be in quite contentment.

Inner Smile Energy Exercise[2]

When we smile we change our relationship to ourselves and to the person, thing or organ we are smiling at. I find the Inner Smile Exercise

---

2   Adapted from Montak *Chia's Chi Self-Massage* (2006). See Bibliography.

to be one of the most powerful exercises for reconnecting with our inner selves. When I am in pain, I send smile energy to my pain. When I am anxious or depressed I send smile energy to my heart. I sometimes stop myself in the middle of the day and just smile into my organs and pay them special respect for working in a well-oiled orchestra.

The Inner Smile is a powerful and healing exercise that uses the energy of happiness and love as a way to communicate with our internal organs and pelvic floor muscles. It increases chi throughout the body. The inner smile begins with the eyes. The eyes are the first organs to receive signals and can cause the organs and glands to accelerate their activity at times of stress or danger. When the eyes are relaxed they activate the parasympathetic nervous system and cause the body to relax. This exercise is a type of inward meditation. Sit in good posture, clasp hands together and breathe deeply.

Imagine you are in one of your most favorite beautiful places in the world. Feel and see all of it in your mind's eye. Now picture the person you love the most there with you. Picture this person smiling at you, and you basking in that love and warmth. Draw this feeling into your eyes.

Picture the healing chi of nature as a golden cloud of benevolent loving energy in front of you.

Draw this energy into your mid-eyebrow point. Feel your eyes and mid-brow area relax as you draw in this beautiful energy. Let this energy amplify the power of your smile.

Smile down into your body and focus on any place that feels tired, sore, painful, weak, empty, or tense. Smile into that area and send love and gratitude into that area.

ADVANCED INNER SMILE:

1. You can go beyond the exercise above and continue the inner smile exercise.

2. Smile into heart and thymus gland and see them open like flowers in the morning with love, joy and happiness. See these feelings bubbling out of them.

3. Smile at your solid organs: lungs, liver, pancreas, spleen, kidneys, sexual organs and reproductive system. Thank them for their work.

4. Smile to your brain, pituitary, thalamus and pineal glands. Then smile at your spinal column going down each vertebrae. Focus on the painful parts of your spine and send the smile energy into them.

5. Finally smile into your navel and collect your energy there. In your **mind's eye** spiral the collected energy outward into a spiral but keep the spiral as small as the size of a grapefruit. We don't want to over-activate any areas so the spiral circles must be kept small and close to the body (about 1 ½ inches). When you need energy smile again at your navel and call upon your energy.

The Goddess Sings Her Song

Many cultures have used sound as a therapeutic tool for thousands of years. Sound healing can be integrated into the mind/body approach to balancing the chakras. You can use the techniques that follow to relieve stress and achieve wellness.

1. **Set the Tone:** Try not to spring out of bed in the morning. Turn to the side, sit up at the side of the bed and do 3 to 5 "Ahhh" tones. While performing these tones, at any pitch, send the intention of gratitude to your heart, thanking your heart for all that it so effortlessly does for you. Imagine your eyes are looking inside your body and bring your gaze down to your heart while doing your tones. Intention is key, so focus on attaching your intention for the day to your tone as you send it into your heart.

2. **Humming:** Any time during the day—in the car, in the morning, when stress arises, before going into an important meeting, etc.—hum any note, any syllable. The key is to hum as softly as you can for as long as you can. Send the vibration of your hum to any place in your body that is holding stress or discomfort. Let the hum fill these areas and unwind the discomfort and stress. (You can even do this with your infants or toddlers on your chest or while holding their hands. They are tied into your heart and the sound of your voice and it will bring relaxation to them as well.) The other goal of humming as long as you can is to practice expelling ALL of the air from your lungs. Most people carry around stagnant air in the lungs for months and months, so this is a good way to re-oxygenate your body. It is very common to yawn until you tear while doing this technique.

3. **Humming with Inner Smile:** Imagine your eyes are able to be removed and turned around so that they are facing inward. Then look down at your body from the inside. Make a small smile and relax your brow as you do your *hummmmm*, any medium note. As softly as you can, as long as you can. Place your hand over your heart and adjust your note until you feel your chest vibrating in your hand. Attach the intention of gratitude to your note and send it to your heart. Thank your heart for all it does, not requesting a day off: "I acknowledge you and I hear you and feel you." Continue to do this exercise until you begin to feel the warmth of your intention and sound filling your heart and warming your hand. If thoughts arise, acknowledge them with lightness and let them know: "Thank you for that, but right now I am acknowledging my heart." Continue to find more air in your lungs and expel the stale air while oxygenating your brain.

4. **Find Your Foundational Note:** Sit comfortably or lie down on a bed or mat. Start with a medium note, any syllable. Sweep the note downward until you reach your comfortable low note. You should be able to tone your low note without any stress to your voice. Once you find your note, chant the tone with the syllable "uuhhh" and visualize your tone and energy going into your perineum. If you are able, you can also perform a *mulabanda* lock while toning and energizing your foundational chakra. Do the same thing going up and use the "eeehhh" vowel at the top of your range. Imagine there is a cord going to the center of the earth on the low note and a cone drawing in energy from the stars on the high note. The up and down energy meets in your heart and radiates out in the front and the back.

5. **Sound Lion with Swan Dive:** When stress from external stimulus or chatter from your left brain brings you into a state of brain imbalance, this technique can quickly dissipate and unwind stress before it gets placed into your body or auric field. If possible, kneel down with your hands on your thighs. Breathe in deeply through the nose and shout out any sound or tone with your mouth open as wide as possible, with your tongue out if possible. Bring your hands out to the side with palms out, stick your chest out, shoulders down, crane your neck back. It is extremely important not to bunch up your shoulders or pinch your neck. You must not create any physical blockages in your body where the stress can get stuck on the way out. Think "swan dive" motion with your body as you tone out your stress. This is also great to do in the car, just remember not to bunch up your body.

6. **Acknowledge Your Left Brain Chatter:** It is not possible to turn off your left brain chatter and thoughts, but it is possible not to let that chatter leave you in a state of fear or paralyzed to move forward. When destructive or crippling thoughts arise,

acknowledge the thoughts with gratitude: they are just trying to help protect you, but at this moment you are not going to act on them. Do not feel anger or hatred toward your thoughts, as this leads to self-hatred and loathing. Send loving gratitude to your thoughts but let them know that right now you want to stay in a state where your left brain and right brain are more in balance.

Whether you have done every exercise in the Goddess Bodywork series or have opted to personalize and strategically choose the massages and techniques that work for you, you have improved your chi and shown yourself self-love. What better way to reclaim your goddess power? With this healing energy radiating through you, you are ready for the next chapter on strategies for keeping your lady parts in their rightful place (prevention and management of pelvic organ prolapse). Let's take a look....

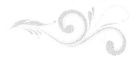

You have come this far, but I have more to teach you.

Energy Medicine That Awakens Your Feminine Sexuality

...to go deeper ONLINE, visit
http://www.FemalePelvicAlchemy.com/chapter9

Energy medicine is no longer standing at the sidelines waiting
to be knowledge. It is a powerful antidote to the stresses of
everyday life and without this type of healing we miss so many
benefits. I have prepared something for you that is very special.
You are going to be so happy after you check this out
that you will probably send me a thank you note☺.
Enjoy the training video.

CHAPTER 10

Keep Your Lady Parts in Their Place

Our female organs are not static. They move and need flexibility for proper functioning. If our organs move too much, lack stability or are not supported as they should be, they can fall out of their proper place and into our vaginas. It sounds scary and there is very little information out there on how we can protect ourselves from having our organs prolapse. So many times I hear new moms, athletes and runners tell me: "If I had only known, I would have protected myself better." So many of my patients get surgeries for organ prolapse only to have them fail or to have complications from the surgery. My advice: before you consider any surgery do the exercises in this book and seek help from a qualified pelvic therapist if needed. Don't get a surgery without first seeking a second and even a third opinion. My program has saved many women from getting surgeries for their prolapses so I am a big believer in doing the work first before going under the knife.

Pelvic organ prolapse, which can be caused by many different factors, can have detrimental effects on a woman's life. I treat women who suffer from organ prolapse after childbirth. Many times I see women with prolapse who are runners or who have an occupation that requires standing for long periods of time. I have often seen women develop pelvic organ prolapse after a bout of bronchitis or chronic coughing. Hormonal status can also affect the organs, and women in menopause can develop prolapse because of decreased estrogen levels. Certain types of surgeries such as hysterectomies also increase the risk for prolapse. Obesity is another risk factor because of the excess weight and pressure that is put on the pelvic floor muscles. Patients with organ prolapse can suffer from symptoms such as pelvic pressure, vaginal bulge, urinary incontinence (UI), fecal incontinence, dyspareunia, constipation, and difficulty emptying both the bladder and bowel. But all is not lost: there are many things you can do naturally to reduce your symptoms, improve the grade of your prolapse and protect yourself from getting one.

Know the Risk Factors Associated with Pelvic Organ Prolapse

First, let's cover risk factors associated with pelvic organ prolapse. Risk factors and causes run the gamut, but we must pay attention to a few key things.

Risk Factors for Organ Prolapse
Diastasis recti abdominal (DRA) separation and poor core strength.
Poor posture, especially anterior tilt pelvis. This posture adds excessive pressure to the anterior wall of the pelvis where the bladder and uterus live.
Impact exercises when you are symptomatic, leaking or in the immediate post-partum period.

Abdominal surgeries, Cesarean births, and mesh surgeries.
Hysterectomies.
Assistive birth: forceps, vacuum or a combination.
Episiotomies or perineal tears.
Constipation and chronic pushing with defecation or urination.
Prolonged second state of labor more than two hours (but could be less).
Breath holding during second stage of labor and directive pushing.
Coccyx injuries or broken coccyx during birth.
Chronic breath holding.
Pregnancy.
Incontinence during pregnancy or in the post-partum period.
Heavy lifting or lifting young child.
Excessive abdominal crunches performed with breath holding and PFM bearing down.
Tight pelvic floor muscles or PFMs that are in spasms.
Pelvic mal-alignment especially sacral posterior torsions.
Herniated disc and low back pain.
Symphysis pubic dysfunction.
Chronic coughing.
Hormonal changes especially a decrease in estrogen.
Multiple pregnancies.
Weight gain

Symptoms of Organ Prolapse
• Sensation of having a ball in the vagina or rectum or a drag-like feeling in the pelvis.
• Pressure in the pelvis.
• Heaviness in the pelvic area.
• A falling-out feeling in the pelvis.
• Rubbing against the underwear contributing to irritation of the vulvar-vaginal area.
• Incontinence: fecal or urinary.
• Gas incontinence or air escaping from the vagina.
• Sexual dysfunction.
• Sexual pain.
• Abdominal pain.
• Low back pain.
• Sacral-iliac pain.
• Feeling like the pelvis is unstable.
• Pain with Kegel exercises.
• Inability to feel complete sensation in the vagina.
• Sexual dysfunction.
• Problems with orgasms.

Goddess's Trade Secrets for Keeping Our Lady Bits in Their Right Place

1. **Train your pelvic floor muscles correctly** and make sure to massage them if they are too tight and/or have too much tension.

2. **Do not push** with defecation or urination because it weakens the muscles and exacerbates pelvic organ symptoms.

3. **Avoid any activity that makes you hold your breath.** Breath holding stresses the pelvic organs and can over time lead to worsening of your prolapse.

4. **Avoid constipation** because it causes you to push and bear down which weakens the pelvic floor muscles, your primary support for your organs.

5. **Use proper potty posture**, which aligns your intestines, urethra and bladder and helps to empty the bowel and bladder without having to push or strain.

6. **Correct your diastasis recti abdominal separation.** When you have an abdominal separation you are at a higher risk for incontinence, organ prolapse, back pain and sexual pain.

7. **Use the resting position at the end of day.** The resting position "unweighs" the pelvis and is simple to do. Place 2 to 3 pillows under your hips so your pelvis is higher than your head. Stay in this position for 20 to 30 minutes. Use at the end of the day to reduce pelvic pressure.

8. **Limit your standing, running and other impact exercises** until your symptoms are under control and your pelvic floor muscles are strong again.

9. **Massage your pelvic floor muscles** so they have normal tension and tone. Pelvic floor muscles that are tight and inflexible will not strengthen as well as pelvic floor muscles that are supple, flexible and have normal tone.

10. **Use the pelvic brace** during strenuous activities, changing positions, laughing, coughing or sneezing. The pelvic brace involves a low-level contraction of your transversus abdominis muscle and your pelvic floor muscles.

11. **Watch your standing posture:** My big trade secret for standing posture is: don't lock your knees. Why? Locking the knees throws you into a swayback posture and increases stress on your joints, bladder and pelvic organs. Bring awareness to how you are standing and correct yourself every time you lock your knees. Keep your knees slightly bent. Another trade secret is to keep your chest lifted and your shoulders pulled back. Imagine that you are wearing a beautiful necklace and you want to show it off to everyone. Keep your head aligned with your neck; avoid forward head posture and keep your chin tucked in. The lower back should be in neutral spine position. Posture is influenced by what we do every day. It may seem easier to stand in poor posture, but at the end of the day your body will not be happy and pain will set in. Poor posture also leads to increased pelvic pressure because the organs are not supported properly. Do yourself a favor and stand up straight.

Please read this book carefully and **create a workout that makes sense for you**.

Prolapse Kegel Program
Goddesses Never Fall Version 1

WHAT TO DO:

1. Lying prone on a physio ball or stool with a resistance band around your legs, turn your toes in toward each other to internally rotate your hips.

2. Perform a Kegel for the recommended length of time while you hold the position. Reverse Kegel as you resume a neutral hip position.

3. Repeat 10 times; perform 3 sets.

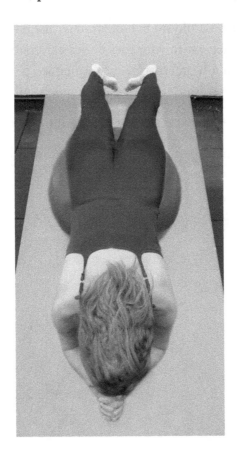

WHAT TO WATCH OUT FOR:

1. Holding your breath, which can increase abdominal pressure and cause leaking, pain, and pressure.

BENEFITS:

1. Strengthens the pelvic floor muscles against gravity.

2. Strengthens the gluteal and hip muscles.

Goddesses Never Fall Version 2

WHAT TO DO:

1. Lying prone on a physio ball or stool with a resistance band around your legs, turn your toes out to externally rotate your hips. Perform a Kegel for the recommended length of time while you hold the position.

2. Reverse Kegel as you resume a neutral hip position.

3. Repeat 10 times; perform 3 sets.

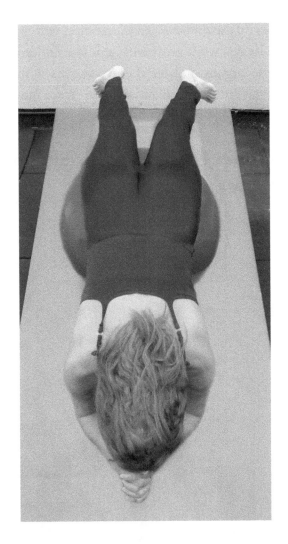

WHAT TO WATCH OUT FOR:

Holding your breath, which can increase abdominal pressure and cause leaking, pain, and pressure.

BENEFITS:

1. Strengthens the pelvic floor muscles against gravity.

2. Strengthens the gluteal and hip muscles.

You can also do the prolapse Kegel exercises with your legs against the wall. These Kegels work great with a pillow underneath the pelvis to "unweigh" the organs and let them come back to their rightful place. These Kegels are powerful and work great for uterine, bladder or rectal prolapse.

Goddesses Never Fall Toe In: Bladder and Uterine Prolapse

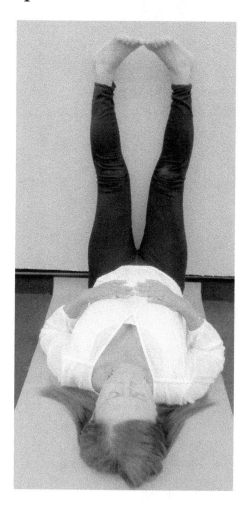

1. Lie on your back and bring buttocks as close to the wall as possible and swing your legs onto wall.

2. Exhale and bring the toes toward each other as you perform your Kegel contraction exercise. Hold for as many seconds as you have determined are right for your program.

3. Inhale and bring your feet to parallel. Perform your reverse Kegel. Then start again. Repeat 5 to 10 times.

Goddesses Never Fall Toe Out: Rectal Prolapse

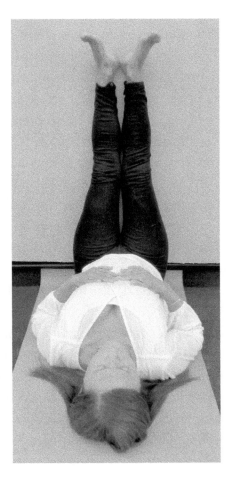

1. Lie on your back and bring buttock as close to the wall as possible and swing your legs onto wall.

2. Exhale and bring your heels together as you perform your Kegel contraction exercise. Hold for as many seconds as you have determined are right for your program.

3. Inhale and bring your feet to parallel. Perform your reverse Kegel exercise. Then start again. Repeat 5 to 10 times.

Another Option: The Pessary

Pessary is a great option for many women suffering from pelvic organ prolapse. This is a device that is inserted into the vagina to support areas of pelvic organ prolapse. Sometimes a woman is too symptomatic and wants to use a pessary until her body gets strong enough for the activities she wants to do. Sometimes I'll recommend a pessary for a woman who has a prolapse and also performs high-level athletic endeavors. In this instance I am looking at the pessary as more of a protection for her pelvic organs and pelvic floor muscles. Pessaries can be life changing and fitting for one is an art form. Even in New York City where I live it is difficult to find a healthcare provider who can fit a pessary with expertise. Many times I find the patient needs to be fitted several times to get it to work properly. So don't be afraid to go back several times for a fitting. A pessary has to fit just right otherwise there is wear and tear on the PFMs, causing them to become tighter and not function as well. It is important to do your alchemical Kegel exercises without the pessary. (NOTE: With some pessaries, it is acceptable to perform Kegels, but double-check with your healthcare provider.)

While a majority of women may note symptom relief with pessary use, some women cannot be successfully fitted, and others may experience burdensome new symptoms during a pessary trial such as discomfort, pressure, or pain. Some may have problems with bowel and bladder emptying, and many complain of an increased vaginal odor. Many can experience new onset stress incontinence due to an inadequately supported urethra. Typically, providers are advised to use caution if pessary candidates have an active vaginal infection, persisting vaginal erosion or ulceration, or severe vaginal atrophy.

Who Should Get One: If you want to avoid a surgery, the pessary is a good option until the PFMs and the core become strong. Check the list below to see who might benefit from a pessary fitting.

1. Pelvic physical therapy is not helping.

2. Cyctocele with symptoms that haven't gotten better with physical therapy.

3. If you are a high-level athlete and want to do high impact exercises or running.

4. Women who are healed from scars in the early post-partum (less than three months post-partum) will benefit from pessary to reduce prolapse and decrease pelvic pressure.

5. You have a uterine prolapse.

6. Prolonged breast feeding and pelvic symptoms are not getting better.

7. If this is a quality-of-life issue you should consider one until you get better with the exercises in this book.

8. Women who are pre-surgical candidates but are not getting pelvic or bladder surgery.

9. Women who have had a hysterectomy, have symptoms, and want to avoid surgeries.

10. Women who have prolapse with either concurrent or latent stress incontinence.

11. Women who have desire for sexual activity but organs are out of the body.

Contraindications and Precautions

There aren't many contraindications, and there are very few precautions when it comes to using a pessary, but you should be aware of what they are.

- Postmenopausal women with thin vaginal mucosa are more susceptible to vaginal ulceration with use of a pessary.

- Active infections of the pelvis or vagina.

- Vaginitis.

- Pelvic inflammatory disease until the infection has been cleared.

- Allergic reaction to material from which the pessary is made. A pessary that is improperly fitted can cause the uterus or cervix to fall through the pessary causing strangulation to those structures, which can lead to necrosis of the cervix or uterus.

- Increased vaginal itching due to the increase in vaginal discharge that is common with pessary usage.

Congratulations, my Queen, my Goddess: You have come back home. You are now poised for a life that is pleasurable, rewarding and ignites your passion. You have returned to your Queendom. My wish for you is that you remember your essence and your beauty and that you stand in your power. Make no excuses, feel everything and release everything. Know that you are enough. For those queens that need and want more, I have developed an extraordinary online companion class, The Female Pelvic Alchemy Online Program. This online workshop contains live videos, community, the female pelvic tracker app, and more transformation. Check it out here:

http://www.pelvicpainrelief.com/femalepelvicalchemy

May the Universe hold you gently in its arms as you remain in your power and in your Queendom.

Big Love,
Isa Herrera

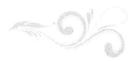

You have come this far, but I have more to teach you.

Keep Your Lady Parts in Their Place

…to go deeper ONLINE, visit
http://www.FemalePelvicAlchemy.com/chapter10

I am so happy that you have reached the end of this book. I truly hope you had a great journey and that you have implemented many of the tools, exercises and techniques that we have explored together. I've saved the best for last: now enjoy the training video for this chapter.

Glossary

Abduction (Hip): Movement of hips away from midline.

Alcock's Canal: A structure within the pelvis through which the pudendal nerve, internal pudendal artery and internal pudendal veins travel. This structure is like a canal formed by the obturator internus fascia.

Annulus Fibrosus: The outer ring of the intervertebral disc made of tough connective tissue. Supports and encases the jelly-like nucleus pulposus.

Anterior Innominate: A pelvic malalignment in which one innominate is rotated anteriorly, or forward, relative to the opposite side.

Anterior Superior Iliac Spine (ASIS): A bony projection on the front of the ilium that serves as an important anatomical landmark.

Biofeedback: Biofeedback training is a nonmedical treatment that helps people improve their health by taking conscious control of their muscles using real-time body signals. Physical therapists use biofeedback to help retrain the pelvic floor muscles.

BMI: Body Mass Index. A formula for determining obesity. An adult with a BMI of 25 to 29.9 is considered overweight, while a BMI of 30 or greater indicates obesity.

Body Mechanics: The way an individual moves his or her body when carrying and lifting objects.

Centralization: Related to low back pain; a process in which distal pain in the lower extremities moves up toward the low back in a more localized area. A sign of improving condition.

Cesarean Section: Incisions are made through the abdominal muscles and uterus to deliver the baby.

Chakra: Chakras are force centers that pulsate subtle energy. Seven major chakras are believed to exist within the body.

Chronic Pelvic Pain: A pelvic pain condition that persists for longer than three months. It is poorly understood and many times requires a multidisciplinary approach for successful treatment.

Coccyx: This bone is found above the anus and in between the gluteal muscles.

Coccyxdynia or Coccygodynia: Pain in the area of the tailbone and its associated structures.

Connective Tissue Rolling (Skin Rolling): A type of massage that is superficial in nature and can be performed on any part of the body, including but not limited to, the abdomen, thighs, buttocks and lower back.

Daily Voiding Log: A diary that helps you track bowel and bladder habits. This tool allows you to quantify urge, leaking, and eating and drinking habits.

Diastasis Recti Abdominis: Separation of rectus abdominis muscles away from the midline that occurs during pregnancy and/or with improper exercise technique and poor body mechanics.

Electrodes: Sensors/pads that can be placed on the body to transmit electrical stimulation with a TENS unit.

Episiotomy: An episiotomy is a surgical incision made at the perineum to enlarge the vagina. This incision can be midline or medial-lateral. It is a common cause of sexual pain and can cause scar tissue in the perineum.

Fascia: A complex web-like system of soft connective tissue that surrounds your organs, muscles, nerves, blood vessels, and other visceral structures and holds your body together. Fascia helps maintain structural integrity, provides support and protection, and acts as a shock absorber.

Gluteus Medius: This is a gluteal muscle that is under the gluteus maximus and can be found to the outside of the butt cheek near the top of the hip bone. This muscle can refer pain to perineum, labia, hip, posterior thigh and sit bone. It can also refer sciatica-like symptoms.

Greater Trochanter of the Femur: This is not a muscle but a very important area that tends to have trigger points and can be a big source of pelvic and hip pain. Many of the posterior hip muscles insert into this bone and it is necessary to reduce or eliminate pain in this area.

Hamstrings: The muscles of the back of the thigh that bend the knee and extend the hip.

Herniated Disc: Extrusion or protrusion of the jelly-like material between bones of the spine; can occur in different degrees and compress surrounding nerves. The inner nucleus pulposus bulge through the tough annulus fibrosus outer ring.

Hip Flexor Muscles: The muscles of the front of the hip that bring the thigh to the trunk.

Homeostasis: A state of balance in the internal environment of the body.

Hypermobility: A condition of excessive flexibility of the joints, allowing them to be bent or moved beyond their normal range of motion.

Hypertension: A condition of abnormally elevated blood pressure.

Hyperthyroidism: A condition of excessive production of thyroid hormones.

Iliac Crest: Prominent bones located at the level of the navel, felt with hands at the waist. The most superior aspect of the innominate bones.

Iliac Crest Line: This is not a muscle but an area where many muscles live. It is the top of hip crest.

Incompetent Cervix: When the cervix dilates before a baby is ready to be born.

Incontinence: Any involuntary leakage or loss of urine.

Innominates: The two bones that form the sides of the pelvis. The innominates are made up of three fused segments: the ilium, ischium and pubis.

Intervertebral Disc: Donut-like structure found between each vertebra of the spine in the cervical, thoracic, and lumbar regions.

It functions as a shock absorber and cushions the spine during activities of daily living. Comprised of a hard outer ring (annulus fibrosus) and jelly-filled inner substance (nucleus pulposus).

Intra-Abdominal Pressure: Pressure within the abdominal cavity.

Isometric Contraction: A type of muscle contraction in which the muscle contracts but does not shorten or change length.

Jackknifing: The act of sitting up straight out of bed; similar to doing a sit-up or crunch.

"Just in Case" (JIC) Urination: This occurs when one urinates out of habit instead of waiting for a proper bladder signal or urinating when the bladder is full. JIC urination is dysfunctional and needs to be eliminated to properly retrain the bladder back to health.

Kegel: An exercise named after Dr. Arnold Kegel that consists of contracting and relaxing the pelvic floor muscles.

L1-L5: L1 through L5 represent the five lumbar spinal vertebrae. The lumbar vertebrae are found between the thoracic and sacral vertebrae in the spinal column. Many times, women with pelvic pain will have some kind of associated dysfunction with L5 and the lumbar spine.

Labia Majora: The outer labia, or outer lips, of the vulva.

Levator Ani Muscles: The muscles that make up the pelvic floor.

Levator Ani Syndrome: Consists of pain, pressure, discomfort or deep dull ache in the vagina and rectum, including the sacrum and coccyx. Levator ani syndrome can also cause burning or radiating pain into the thighs and buttocks. Pain with sitting and defecation are common complaints. Many times the pelvic floor muscles are in spasms and have multiple trigger points in them.

Ligaments: Ligaments are structures that hold bones together and prevent excessive movement of the joint.

Lithotomy: Common position for childbirth and gynecologic/pelvic exam; lying flat on back, with feet above or level with hips.

Lumbar Lordosis: The natural curvature of the lower spine in a slightly arched posture. Also known as the "sway back" posture, it can become excessive during pregnancy.

Lumbar Shift: A compensation seen with low back pain in which the upper body shifts away from the lower body in order to take pressure off of a painful segment in the low back.

Lumbar Spine: The segment of the human spine above the pelvis and below the ribs that is involved in low back pain. There are five vertebrae, or bones, in the lumbar spine.

Muscle Energy Technique (MET): MET is an osteopathic technique that involves gentle muscle contraction performed against gentle resistance in a specific direction.

Myofascial Release: This is a connective tissue hands-on therapy for the treatment of muscle pain and immobility.

Neutral Spine (NS): Neutral spine is the natural position of the spine when all the parts of the spine—cervical, thoracic and lumbar—are in excellent alignment.

Nucleus Pulposus: Jelly-like center of the intervertebral disc made mostly of water, which acts as the cushioning support of the spine.

Obturator Internus Muscle: The obturator internus muscle is found within the pelvis and within the hip-joint. This muscle helps to externally rotate the leg, extend the thigh and abduct the flexed thigh. It also helps to stabilize femoral head in the acetabulum.

This muscle can cause sexual pain, hip pain and/or a deep ache in the pelvis. The obturator internus can refer pain to anywhere within the pelvic girdle. This muscle can be accessed through the vagina and rectum and can frequently have spasms and trigger points causing sexual and pelvic pain.

Osteopathic: Osteopathic techniques use the hands, rather than machinery, to diagnose, treat and prevent injury.

Pelvic Floor: A complex set of muscles, nerves and connective tissue that form the cradle or basket of your being.

Pelvic Floor Muscle Dysfunction: Abnormal or impaired function of the pelvic floor muscles.

Pelvic Floor Muscle Hypertonicity: Muscular hypertonicity is a disorder in which muscles continually receive a message to tighten and to contract. This causes excessive stiffness or tightness and interferes with their normal function.

Pelvic Floor Muscle Incoordination: A lack of normal and harmonious muscle action in the pelvic floor muscles.

Pelvic Floor Muscle Spasm: Involuntary contraction of a pelvic floor muscle.

Pelvic Floor Muscles: The pelvic floor muscles consist of three layers of muscle that support your pelvis, control urination and defecation and allow for optimal sexual function.

Pelvic Girdle: The pelvic girdle is the bony ring that makes up the human pelvis. The pelvic girdle consists of two innominates and one sacrum.

Pelvic Release: A lengthening release of the pelvic floor muscles that can be performed with either inhalation or exhalation.

Perineal Body: The central area between the rectum and the vagina in the perineum. It is also the area where most of the pelvic floor muscles are attached.

Perineal Tearing: Tears to the perineum (the area between the genitalia and anus) that can cause damage to the anal sphincter causing fecal incontinence, urgency, pain during intercourse or other problems.

Perineal Tears in Degrees: Tears are rated from 1st to 4th Degree. 1st Degree is tearing of the vaginal mucosa skin at or around the perineal body. 2nd Degree is tearing vaginal mucosa and submucosa through the pelvic floor muscles. 3rd Degree is tearing of the 1st and 2nd Degree tissues and the external sphincter. 4th Degree is all of the above levels of tearing plus the internal sphincter and the lining of the rectum.

Perineum: The diamond-shaped area between the legs that houses muscles and rectum, and in females, includes the vagina. This can also refer to both the superficial or deep structures in this region.

Peripheralization: Related to low back pain; a process by which pain in the low back spreads or radiates into the lower extremities. A sign of worsening condition.

Piriformis Syndrome: A disorder that occurs when the sciatic nerve is compressed, pinched or irritated by the piriformis muscle. This compression can cause pain, tingling and numbness in the buttocks and along the sciatic nerve path.

Posterior Innominate: A pelvic malalignment in which one innominate is rotated posteriorly, or backward, relative to the opposite side.

Posterior Superior Iliac Spine (PSIS): Bony prominence on each hip bone palpable where the "dimples" in the lower back can be found on many men and women.

Preterm Labor: Labor that occurs before the thirty-seventh week of pregnancy.

Prolapse: An organ moves down into and protrudes through the vaginal canal or anal opening, resulting in the sensation of pressure or visible protrusion. The uterus, rectum, bladder or urethra can prolapse into the vagina and cause pelvic floor muscle weakness.

Psoas Muscle: This is deep muscle that cannot be seen from the outside of the body. It comes from lumbar spine and inserts into the top of the leg bone. This muscle can be a source of pelvic pain and many times has trigger points in it that refer pain to the hip, low back and vulvar-vaginal area.

Pubic Bone: This bone forms the anterior aspect of the pelvis and hip bones.

Pubic Symphysis: Cartilaginous joint located between two pubic bones, connects the two pelvis bones.

Pudendal Nerve: This nerve arises from the ventral rami of nerve roots S2 to S4 and from the pudendal nerve trunk. The pudendal nerve is a mix nerve with sensory, motor and autonomic fibers. It has three terminal branches that include dorsal nerve of the clitoris, perineal branch and inferior rectal branch. The pudendal nerve is the main nerve of the perineum and supplies the PFMs, vagina, urethra, skin of labia, external anal sphincter, urethral sphincter, anal canal, anal skin, clitoris and sensory to the lower vagina. Sometimes this nerve can be injured in childbirth.

Pudendal Nerve Neuralgia (PNN): A shooting, stabbing and knife-like pain that can occur anywhere in the distribution of the pudendal nerve. Some women experience this kind of condition after childbirth.

Quadratus Lumborum: This muscle can be found posterior in between the lower ribs and the top of the hip bone but lateral to the paraspinal muscles. Once you are in this area you have to press in toward the spine to find the trigger point. This muscle can be a big pelvic pain generator and must be addressed.

Rectus Abdominis: This is the six-pack abdominal muscle; it runs from below the breast bone to the pubic bone. There are two sides, one to the right of the belly button and one to the left that are connective via the linea alba. A separation of this muscle at the linea alba is called diastasis recti.

Reverse Kegel: This exercise is an elongation and relaxation exercise for the PFMs.

Round Ligament: Ligament that connects the uterus to the groin, often stretched in pregnancy and a common site of pain.

Round Ligament Pain: A sharp, stabbing pain that occurs due to a sudden tightening of a ligament that travels from the uterus to the labia majora.

Rupture of Membranes: Rupture of amniotic sac, commonly referred to as "water breaking" that occurs before the baby is delivered.

S2-S5: S2 through S5 are vertebrae of the sacral spine. The sacral spine is below the lumbar spine and is located at the base of the spine.

Sacral Torsion: A sacral torsion is a rotation of the sacrum that disrupts the normal mechanics of the SI joint.

Sacroiliac (SI) Joint: The joint formed in the back of the pelvis by the sacrum and innominates. This joint is often a source of pain during pregnancy due to misalignment, hypermobility and muscle weakness.

Sacrum: The sacrum is a triangular-shaped bone that forms the back of the pelvis; it is inserted like a wedge between the two hip bones. Its upper edge connects to the last lumbar vertebra, and its bottom connects with the coccyx (tailbone). The sacral nerves exit through small holes in the sacrum.

Scar: A scar is part of the natural healing process of wound repair in the skin and other tissues of the body.

Sciatic: Relating to the nerve roots that come from the spinal cord, forming a bundle of nerves that travel down the legs, passing beneath the muscles, where they can become compressed and cause pain.

Sciatica: Irritation to the sciatic nerve in the low back or buttock region causing pain, numbness, and/or tingling into the lower extremities.

Shotgun Correction: The shotgun correction is a pelvic MET that aligns the joint of the pubic symphysis.

Sit Bones: Also called ischial tuberosity, sit bones are the bones that we sit on. These bones have surrounding fascia that are intimately connected with the gluteal and hip muscles. Many times women suffering from pelvic pain experience pain at these bones. The gluteal muscles, adductor muscles, PFMs and PNN can refer pain to the sit bones. An exhaustive investigation is required to find out the exact cause of sit bone pain.

Skin Rolling: Also know as connective tissue rolling, this is a type of massage used for releasing and clearing barriers, fascial restrictions and trigger points in muscles.

Stress Incontinence: Urinary leakage that occurs as a result of pressure on the bladder with changing positions, coughing, laughing, sneezing, lifting or exercise.

Supine Hypotension: A drop in blood pressure that can occur when a pregnant woman is lying on her back.

Symphysis Pubis Dysfunction: A painful condition that is caused by excessive movement in the pubic symphysis joint.

Tendinous Arch of the Levator Ani: A thickened portion of the obturator fascia where some of the levator ani muscles originate. This fascia can be painful to the touch. Let an experienced PT show you how to correctly release this fascia.

TENS (Transcutaneous Electrical Nerve Stimulation) Unit: A unit used to deliver electrical stimulation to the skin for pain relief.

Tension Release Breathing (TRB): A breathing technique—coined by author Isa Herrera—using mind/body connection to release pain and tension of a painful muscle. The individual inhales into the painful body part while thinking about collecting her pain as she inhales. Then the individual exhales and visualizes the pain leaving her body. This type of breathing should be performed for five breaths.

Thorax: Central region of the body which is partially encased by the rib cage and contains many vital organs such as the heart and lungs.

Transverse Abdominis Muscle: The innermost, deepest abdominal muscle that acts like a "corset" and provides significant stability to the trunk when activated appropriately. It has an intimate relationship with the PFMs.

"Tucked Tush" Posture: Decreased lumbar lordosis, or flattened low back, caused by shortening of the gluteal muscles and shift in center of gravity during pregnancy.

Type 1 Diabetes: Common in children and younger individuals; a condition in which the body does not produce insulin, resulting in increased blood glucose levels.

Urge Incontinence: Urinary leakage that occurs following a sudden, intense urge to urinate.

Urgency or Frequency of Urination: Frequent urination (urinating at intervals less than three to four hours, or more than eight voids per day) or urgency of urination without an increase in the total urine held in the bladder. This condition may result from infections, a small bladder capacity, other structural abnormalities, from food irritants, or trigger points.

Uterosacral Ligaments: Ligaments that connect the uterus to the sacrum. When the sacrum is not in proper alignment, these ligaments may affect the position of the uterus.

Valsalva Maneuver: A forced exhalation where breath is held and air does not leave the body, resulting in increased pressure in the abdominal cavity.

Varicosity: Swollen, painful veins.

Vertebrae: The bones that form the spinal column.

Vertex Position: The vertex position describes a fetus that is head-down prior to birth.

Vulvodynia, Provoked: A type of vulvodynia that occurs with direct contact with the vulva.

Vulvodynia, Unprovoked: A type of vulvodynia that causes vulvar pain, burning, and discomfort without direct contact to the vulvar area.

Bibliography

Abbott, J. (2009). Gynecological indications for the use of botulinum toxin in women with chronic pelvic pain. *Toxicon.* 2009 Oct; 54(5):647-53. Epub 2009 Mar 3.

Abbott, J., Jarvis, S., Lyons, S., Thomson, A., & Vancaille, T. (2006). Botulinum toxin type A for chronic pain and pelvic floor spasm in women: a randomized controlled trial. *Obstetrics & Gynecology,* 108(4), 915-923.

Abraham, K. (2002). A special update on chronic pelvic pain from the conference: Chronic pelvic pain: Pathogenic mechanisms, treatment, innovations, and research implications. *Journal of the Section on Women's Health,* 26(3), 9-12.

Albert, H., Godskesen, M., Westergaard, J. (1999). Evaluation of clinical tests used in classification procedures in pregnancy-related pelvic joint pain. *European Spine Journal,* 9(2) 161-166.

Alcantara, Margarita. (2017). *Chakra Healing: A Beginner's Guide to Self-Healing Techniques That Balance the Chakras.* Berkeley, CA: Althea Press.

Arvigo, Rosita, and Epstein, Nadine. (2001). *Rainforest Remedies: The Maya Way to Heal Your Body & Replenish Your Soul*. New York, NY: Harper Collins Publishers.

Barber, M.D., Walters, M.D., Bump, R.C. Short forms of two condition-specific quality-of-life questionnaires for women with pelvic floor disorders (PFDI-20 adn PFIQ-7). *Am J Obstet Gynecol* 2005; 193:103-113.

Barral, Jean-Pierre. (1993). *Urogenital Manipulation*. Seattle, WA: Eastland Press.

Barral, Jean-Pierre. (1989). *Visceral Manipulation*. Seattle, WA: Eastland Press.

Barral, Jean-Pierre. (2007). *Visceral Manipulation II (Revised Edition)*. Seattle, WA: Eastland Press.

Barral, Jean-Pierre, and Kuchera, Michael L. (2007). *Visceral and Obstetric Osteopathy*. Edinburgh, England: Churchill Livingstone.

Barral, Jean-Pierre and Mercier, Pierre. (2005). *Visceral Manipulation, Revised Edition*. Seattle, WA: Eastland Press.

Barral, Jean-Pierre, DO, Wetzler, Gail, RPT, Ahern, Dee, RPT, Grant, Lisa Brady, DC. (2005). *Visceral Manipulation: Abdomen 2 Study Guide*. West Palm Beach, FL: The Barral Institute.

Barral, Jean-Pierre, DO, Wetzler, Gail, RPT. (2005). *Visceral Manipulation: Abdomen 1 Study Guide*. West Palm Beach, FL: The Barral Institute.

Beco, Jacques. (2001). Relevant Anatomy of Pudendal Nerve and Etiological Factors of Pudendal Neuropathies. Retrieved February 18, 2014 from http://www.perineology.com/files/ics-glasgow-anatomy.pdf.

Bergeron, S., et al. (2001). Vulvar vestibular syndrome: Reliability of diagnosis and evaluation of current diagnostic criteria. *Obstet Gynecol.* Vol. 98, 45-51.

Bergeron, S., Binik, Y. M., Khalifé, S., Pagidas, K., & Glazer, H. I. (2001). Vulvar vestibular syndrome: Rehabilitation of diagnosis and evaluation of current diagnostic criteria. *Obstetrics & Gynecology,* 98(1), 45-51.

Berghmans, L. C., Hendriks, H. J., Bo, K., Hay-Smith, E. J., de Bie, R. A., & van Waalwijk van Doorn, E. S. (1998). Conservative treatment of stress urinary incontinence in women: A systematic review of randomized clinical trials. *British Journal of Urology,* 82(2), 181-91.

Berghmans, L., Frederiks, C., de Bie, R., Weil, E., Smeets, L., van Waalwijk van Doorn, E., et al. (1996). Efficacy of biofeedback, when included with pelvic floor muscle exercise treatment, for genuine stress incontinence. *Neurology and Urodynamics,* 15(1), 37-52.

Block, Jennifer. (2007). *Pushed:. The Painful Truth about Childbirth and Modern Maternity Care.* Cambridge, MA: Da Capo Press.

Bo, Kari, Berghmans, Bary, Morkved, Siv, Van Kampen, Marijke. (2007). *Evidence-Based Physical Therapy for the Pelvic Floor.* London: Churchill Livingstone, Elsevier Health Sciences.

Bo, K., & Sherburn, M. (2005). Evaluation of female pelvic floor muscle function and strength. *Physical Therapy,* 85(3), 269-282.

Borello-France, D., Zyczynski, H., Downey, P, Rause, C. & Wister, J. (2006). Effect of pelvic-floor muscle exercise position on continence and quality-of-life outcomes in women with stress urinary incontinence. *Physical Therapy,* 86(7), 974-986.

Bouchez, Colette. (2001). *The V Zone: A Woman's Guide to Intimate HealthCare*. New York, NY: Fireside.

Brennan, Barbara. (1988). *Hands of Light: A Guide to Healing Through the Human Energy Field*. New York, NY: Bantam Books.

Brennan, Barbara. (1993). *Light Emerging: The Journey of Personal Healing Bantam Books*. New York, NY: Bantam Books.

Butler, D. S. (2004). *Mobilisation of the Nervous System*. Edinborough: Churchill Livingston.

Calais-Germain, Blandine. (2005). *Anatomy of Breathing*. Seattle, WA: Eastland Press.

Calais-Germain, Blandine. (2003). *The Female Pelvis: Anatomy & Exercises*. Seattle, WA: Eastland Press.

Calleja-Agius J, Brincat MP. (2009). Urogenital atrophy. *Climacteric*. Apr 22, pp. 1-7.

Carriere, Neate, and Feldt, Cynthia Markel. (2006). *The Pelvic Floor*. Stuttgart, Germany: Georg Thieme Verlag.

Cauthery, Dr. Philip, Stanway, Dr. Andrew, and Stanway, Dr. Penny. (1983). *The Complete Book of Love and Sex*. Great Britain: Century Publishing Co. Ltd.

Chaitow, Leon, Lovegrove Jones, Ruth. (2012). *Chronic Pelvic Pain and Dysfunction: Practical Physical Medicine*. London: Churchill Livingstone, Elsevier Health Sciences.

Chaitow, Leon. (2006). *Muscle Energy Techniques*. London: Churchill Livingstone, Elsevier Health Sciences.

Chaitow, Leon. (2007). *Positional Release Techniques*. London: Churchill Livingstone, Elsevier Health Sciences.

Chia, Mantak. (2006). *Chia Self-Massage: The Taoist Way of Rejuvenation*. Rochester, VT: Destiny Books.

Chia, Mantak. (2008). *Healing Light of the Tao*. Rochester, VT: Destiny Books.

Chu, K. K., Chen, F. P., Chang, S. D., & Soong, Y. K. (1995). Laparoscopic presacral neurectomy in the treatment of dysmenorrhea. *Diagnostic and Therapeutic Endoscopy*, 1, 223-225.

Coccydynia. (n.d.). In Wikipedia. Retrieved March 10, 2014 from http://en.wikipedia.org/wiki/Coccydynia.

D'Amborosio, Kerry J, Roth, George B. (1997). *Positional Release Therapy, Assessment and Treatment of Musculoskeletal Dysfunction*. St. Louis, MO: Mosby.

Davies, Clair and Amber Davies. (2004). *The Trigger Point Therapy Workbook: Your Self-Treatment Guide for Pain Relief*. Oakland, CA: New Harbinger Publications.

Davis, Martha, Ph.D, Robbins-Eshelman, Elizabeth, M.S.W., and McKay, Matthew, Ph.D. (2000). *The Relaxation and Stress Reduction Workbook*. New York, NY: MJM Books.

Dell, JR, Mokrzycki, ML, Jayne, CJ. (2009). Differentiating interstitial cystitis from similar conditions commonly seen in gynecologic practice. *Eur J Obstet Gynecol Reprod Biol*. Apr 29.

Derry, DE. (1907). Pelvic muscles and fasciae. *Journal of Anatomy and Physiology*, 42:107-11.

Drake, Richard L., Vogl, A. Wayne, Mitchell, Adam W.M., Tibbitts, Richard M., Richardson, Paul E. (2008). *Gray's Atlas of Anatomy*. London: Churchill Livingstone, Elsevier Health Sciences.

Dul, Jan and Weerdmeester, Bernard. (2001). *Ergonomics for Beginners: A Quick Reference Guide. Second Edition.* London: Taylor & Francis.

Dumoulin, C., Lemieux, M., Bourbonnais, D., Gravel, D., Bravo, G. & Morin, M. (2004). Physiotherapy for persistent postnatal stress urinary incontinence: a randomized controlled trial. *Obstetrics & Gynecology,* 104(3), 504-510.

Dye, J. (2004). Fertility of American Women: June 2004. *Current Population Report,* December 2005, 1-14.

Ehrstrom S, Kornfeld D, Rylander E, Bohm-Starke N. (2009). Chronic stress in women with localized provoked vulvodynia. *J Psychosom Obstet Gynaecol.* March Vol. 30(1), pp. 73-9.

Epstein, Abby, and Lake, Ricki. (2009). *Your Best Birth.* New York, NY: Hachette Book Group.

Erekson, E. A., Yip, S. O., Wedderburn, T. S., Martin, D. K., Li, F.-Y., Choi, J. N., Kenton, K.S., Fried, T. R. (2013). The VSQ: a questionnaire to measure vulvovaginal symptoms in postmenopausal women. *Menopause (New York, N.Y.), 20*(9), 973–979. http://doi.org/10.1097/GME.0b013e318282600b.

Fanucci E, Manenti G, Ursone A, Fusco N, Mylonakou I, D'Urso S, Simonetti G. (2009). Role of interventional radiology in pudendal neuralgia: a description of techniques and review of the literature. *Radiol Med.* Mar 10.

Fisher, K. & Riolo, L. (2004). Evidence in practice. *American Physical Therapy Association Inc.* Retrieved June 12, 2008 from http://www.thefreelibrary.com/evidence+in+practice-a0120610455.com.

FitzGerald, M.P. & Kotarinos, R. (2003). Rehabilitation of the short pelvic floor. I: Background and patient evaluation. *International Urogynecological Journal,* 14(4), 261-268.

FitzGerald, M.P. & Kotarinos, R. (2003). Rehabilitation of the short pelvic floor, II: Treatment of the patient with the short pelvic floor. *International Urogynecological Journal,* 14 (4), 269-275.

Foye, Patrick, & Buttacci, Charles. (2012). Coccyx Pain. *In Medscape.* Retrieved March 10, 2014 from http://emedicine.medscape. com/article/309486- overview#aw2aab6b2b2.

Foye, Patrick, & Buttacci, Charles. (2012). Coccyx Pain Treatment & Management. *In Medscape.* Retrieved March 12, 2014 from http://emedicine.medscape.com/article/309486- treatment#aw2aab6b6b3.

Franklin, Eric. (2002). *Pelvic Power: Mind/Body Exercises for Strength, Flexibility, Posture, and Balance.* Hightstown, NJ: Princeton Book Company.

Gach, Michale Reed. (1990). *Acupressure's Potent Points.* New York, NY: Bantam Books.

Gerwin, R., Dommerholt, J., & Shah, J. (2004). An explanation of simons' integrated hypothesis of trigger point formation. *Current Science Inc.,* 8, 468-475.

Gilroy, Anne M., MacPherson, Brian R., Ross, Lawrence M. (2008). *Atlas of Anatomy (1st ed).* New York, NY: Thieme Medical Publishers, Inc.

Glazer, H., & MacConkey, D. (1996). Functional rehabilitation of pelvic floor muscles: A challenge to tradition. Urologic Nursing, 16, 68-9. Retrieved May 25, 2008 from http://www.vulvodynia. com/fropfm.htm.

Goldberg, Roger. (2003). *Ever Since I Had My Baby: Understanding, Treating, and Preventing the Most Common Physical Aftereffects of Pregnancy and Childbirth.* New York, NY: Three Rivers Press.

Goldfinger C., Pukall CF., Gentilcore-Saulnier E., McLean L., Chamberlain S. (2009). A prospective study of pelvic floor physical therapy: Pain and psychosexual outcomes in provoked vestibulodynia. *J Sex Med.* April 28.

Goldstein, A. (2008). Vulvodynia (CME). *J Sex Med.* 2008 Jan;5 (1):5-15 18173761. Retrieved December 12, 2008, from http:// lib.bioinfo.pl/auth:Goldstein,AT.

Goldstein, A. (2007). New diagnosis for vestibular pain and redness: Don't get lumped in a general category again! *OurGyn.* Retrieved February 12, 2009, from http://www.ourgyn.com.

Goldstein, A. (2007). Vaginal pain and itching with no known cause? *OurGyn.* Retrieved February 21, 2009, from http://www.ourgyn. com.

Goldstein, A. (2007). 14 different treatments for vulvar vestibulitis syndrome. *OurGyn.* Retrieved May 23, 2008 from http://www.ourgyn.com/content/index.php?option=com_ content&task=view&id=18&Itemid=66.

Goldfinger, S. (2007). Gas and bloating. *UpToDate.* Retrieved July 11, 2008, from http://www.uptodate.com/patients/content/topic. do?topicKey=~ S6QjVerp-W9eT4.

Gustafson, KJ, Zelkovic, PF, Feng, AH, Draper, CE, Bodner, DR, Grill, WM. (2005). Fascicular anatomy and surgical access of the human pudendal nerve. *World J Urol.* 2005 Dec; 23(6):411-8. Epub 2005 Dec 7. Retrieved February 10, 2014 from http:// www.ncbi.nlm.nih.gov/pubmed/16333625.

Haefner, H., Collins, M., Davis, G., Edwards, L., Foster, D., Hartmann, E., et al (2005). The Vulvodynia Guideline. *Journal of Lower Genital Tract Disease*, 9(1), 40-51.

Harlow, B., & Stewart, E. (2003). A population-based assessment of chronic unexplained vulvar pain: Have we underestimated the prevalence of vulvodynia? *Journal of the American Medical Women's Association*, 58(2), 82-87.

Haslam, Jeanette, and Laycock, Jo. (2002). *Therapeutic Management of Incontinence and Pelvic Pain. Second Edition*. London, England: Springer-Verlag.

Hay, Louise L. (1999). *You Can Heal Your Life*. Carlsbad, CA: Hay House Inc.

Hopwood, Val, and Lovesey, Maureen, and Mokone, Sara. (1997). *Acupuncture & Related Techniques in Physical Therapy*. Edinburgh, England: Churchill Livingstone.

Hruby S, Ebmer J, Dellon AL, Aszmann, OC. (2005). Anatomy of the pudendal nerve at the urogenital diaphragm: A new critical site for nerve entrapment, *Urology*, 66: 949-952.

Hulme, Janet A. (1997). *Beyond Kegels. Second Edition*. Missoula, MT: Phoenix Publishing Co.

Hummel-Berry, K., Wallace, K., Herman, H. *Vulvar Pain Functional Questionnaire*. 2005.

Hutcherson, Hilda. (2002). *What Your Mother Never Told You About S-e-x*. New York, NY: Berkley Publishing Group.

Ischioanal Fossa. (2013, June 20). Retrieved February 4, 2014 from the Wiki: http://en.wikipedia.org/wiki/Ischioanal_fossa.

Jones, L. H., Kusunose, R. H. & Goering, E. K. (1995). *Jones Strain-Counterstrain*. Boise, ID: Jones Strain-Counterstrain Inc.

Kabatt-Zin, Jon. (2005). *Coming to Our Senses*. New York, NY: Hyperion.

Kashefi F, Khajehei M, Ashraf AR, Jafari P. (2011). The efficacy of acupressure at the Sanyinjiao point in the improvement of women's general health. *J Altern Complement Med.* Dec; 17(12):1141-7. Epub 2011 Nov 14.

Katz, Ditza and Ross Lynn Tabisel. (2005). *Private Pain: Understanding Vaginismus & Dyspareunia. Second Edition.* Canada: Katz-Tabi Publications.

Kavaler, Elizabeth. (2006). *A Seat on the Aisle, Please: The Essential Guide to Urinary Tract Problems in Women*. New York, NY: Copernicus Books.

Kellogg-Spadt, S., & Albaugh, J. (2002). Intimacy and bladder pain: helping women reclaim sexuality. *Urologic Nursing*, 22(5), 355-56.

Kellogg-Spadt, S., & Giordano, J. (2002). Vulvar Vestibulitis and Sexual Pain. *The Female Patient*, 27, 51-53.

Klein, M., & Robbins, R. (1998). *Let Me Count the Ways: Discovering Great Sex Without Intercourse*. New York, NY: Penguin Putnam Inc.

KMom (2003). Pelvic pain (Symphysis publis dysfunction). Retrieved August 14, 2008, from http://www.plus-size-pregnancy.org/pubicpain.htm.

Kolster, B. C., Waskowiak, A., & Myint, N. W. (2007). *The Acupressure Atlas (1st U.S. ed.)*. Rochester, VT: Healing Arts Press.

Lachowsky M, Nappi R. (2009). The effects of estrogen on urogenital health. *Maturitas*. April 30.

Lee, R. B., Stone, K., Magelssen, D., Belts, R. P., & Benson, W. L. (1986). Presacral neurectomy for chronic pelvic pain. *Obstetrics & Gynecology*, 68, 517- 521. Retrieved April 17, 2008, from http://www.greenjournal.org/cgi/content/abstract/68/4/517.

Levin-Gervasi, Stephanie. (1995). *The Back Pain Sourcebook*. Los Angeles, CA: Lowell House.

Lundberg, Paul. (2003). *The Book of Shiatsu*. New York, NY: Simon and Schuster.

Magee, David J. (2002). *Orthopedic Physical Assessment*. Philadelphia, PA: Saunders Publications.

Maigne, Jean-Yves. (2002). *Management of Common Coccygodynia*. Retrieved February 1, 2014 from http://www.coccyx.org/medabs/maigne6.htm.

Makichen, Walter. (2005). *Spirit Babies. How to Communicate with the Child You're Meant to Have*. New York, NY: Bantam Dell.

Manheim, Carol. (2001). *The Myofascial Release Manual. Third Edition*. Thorofare, NJ: Slack Inc.

Mercier, Patricia. (2007). *The Chakra Bible*. New York, NY: Sterling Publishing.

Miller, P., Forstein, D. & Styles, S. (2008). Effect of short-term diet and exercise on hormone levels and menses in obese, infertile women. *Journal of Reproductive Medicine*, 53(5), 315-319.

Mojay, Gabriel. (1997). *Aromatherapy for Healing the Spirit: Restoring Emotional and Mental Balance with Essential Oils*. Rochester, VT: Healing Arts Press.

Moldwin, R. (2000). *The Interstitial Cystitis Survival Guide: Your Guide to the Latest Treatment Options and Coping Strategies.* Oakland, CA: New Harbinger Publications.

Morkved, S., Bo, K. & Fjortoft, T. (2002). Effect of adding biofeedback to pelvic floor muscle training to treat urodynamic stress incontinence. *Obstetrics & Gynecology,* 100(4), 730-739.

Myers, Thomas W. (2001). *Anatomy Trains. Myofascial Meridians and Movement Therapists.* Edinburgh, England: Churchill Livingstone.

Netter, Frank H. (1997). *Atlas of Human Anatomy (4th ed).* Teterboro, NJ: Icon Learning Systems.

Neumann, Donald A. (2002). *Kinesiology of the Musculoskeletal System: Foundations or Physical Rehabilitation(1st ed).* St. Louis: Mosby Inc.

Newman, D. (2008). Understanding electrical stimulation as a treatment for incontinence. *Seekwellness.* Retrieved January 14, 2009, from http://www.seekwellness.com/incontinence/electric_stim.htm.

Noble, Elizabeth. (1995). *Essential Exercises for the Childbearing Year.* Harwich, MA: New Life Images.

Paoletti, Serge. (2006). *The Fasciae Anatomy, Dysfunction and Treatment.* Seattle, WA: Eastland Press.

Pelvic Health Solutions: Active Pudendal Nerve Gliding. Retrieved February 1, 2014 from http://www.pelvichealthsolutions.ca/for-the-patient/pudendal-nerve-irritation/neural-tension/.

Prendergast, S., & Weiss, J. (2003). Screening for musculoskeletal causes of pelvic pain. *Clinical Obstetrics & Gynecology,* 46(4), 1-10.

Prendergast, S. How do I know if I have PN or PNE? *Pelvic Health and Rehabilitation Center.* Retrieved January 14, 2014 http://www.pelvicpainrehab.com/pelvic-pain/726/how-do-i-know-if-i-have-pn-or-pne/.

Rao, S. (2004). Diagnosis and management of fecal incontinence. *The American Journal of Gastroenterology*, 99(8), 1585-1604.

Reninger, Elizabeth. (2017). Acupressure Treasures: Bai Hui - Hundred Convergences. Retrieved May 4, 2017 from Thought Co: https://www.thoughtco.com/acupressure-treasures-bai-hui-hundred-convergences-3182275.

Rogers, Rebecca G, Janet Yagoda Shagam and Shelley Kleinschmidt. (2006). *Regaining Bladder Control: What Every Woman Needs to Know.* New York, NY: Prometheus Books.

Sahrmann, A. Shirley. (2002). *Diagnosis and Treatment of Movement Impairment Syndromes.* St. Louis: Mosby Inc.

Sapsford, R., & Hodges, P. (2001). Contraction of the pelvic floor muscles during abdominal maneuvers. *Archives of Physical Medicine and Rehabilitation*, 82(8), 1081-8.

Sapsford Aua, Ruth et al. (1998). *Women's Health: A Textbook for Physiotherapists.* New York: WB Saunders Company Ltd.

Sapsford, R. (2001). "Contraction of the pelvic floor muscles during abdominal maneuvers." Abstract: *Arch Phys Med Rehabil.* Vol. 81, 1081-8.

Schnaubet, Kurt. (1999). *Medical Aromatherapy. Healing with Essential Oils.* Berkely, CA: Frog, Ltd.

Shamliyan, T., Kane, R., Wyman, J. & Wilt, T. (2008). Systematic review: randomized, controlled trials of nonsurgical treatments for urinary incontinence in women. *Annals of Internal Medicine*, 148(6), 459-473.

Spadt-Kellogg, S.,et al. (2002). Vulvar vestibulitis and sexual pain: New insights. *The Female Patient*. Vol. 27, 51-53.

Spadt-Kellogg, Susan, et al. (2002). Intimacy and bladder pain: Helping women reclaim sexuality. *Urologic Nursing* Vol. 22:5, 355-56.

Spatafora, Denise. (2009). *Better Birth*. Hoboken, NJ: Wiley and Sons, Inc.

Steege JF, Zolnoun DA. (2009). Evaluation and treatment of dyspareunia. *Obstet Gynecol*. May 113(5), pp. 1124-36.

Stewart, Elizabeth G. and Paula Spencer. (2002). *The V Book: A Doctor's Guide to Complete Vulvovaginal Health*. New York, NY: Bantam Books.

Sutton KS, Pukall CF, Chamberlain S. (2009). Pain ratings, sensory thresholds, and psychosocial functioning in women with provoked vestibulodynia. *J Sex Marital Ther*. Vol. 35(4), pp. 262-81.

Tjaden, B., Schlaff, W. D., Kimball, A., & Rock, J. A. (1990). The efficacy of presacral neurectomy for the relief of midline dysmenorrhea. Obstetrics & Gynecology, 76, 89-91. Retrieved February 13, 2008, from http://www.greenjournal.org/cgi/content/abstract/76/1/89.

Tolle, Eckhart. (1999). *The Power of Now*. Vancouver, Canada: Namaste Publishing.

Traditional Chinese Medicine: Distribution of the Twelve Meridians. Retrieved May 4, 2017, from http://www.shen-nong.com/eng/principles/distributionmeridians.html.

Urogenital Diaphragm and Ishiorectal Fossa. (2006, March 30). Retrieved from http://download.videohelp.com/vitualis/med/urogenital_diaphragm_ischiorectal_fossa.ht.

Wallace, Kathe and Holly Herman. (2006). *Female Pelvic Floor: Function, Dysfunction and Treatment. Level 2B.* The Prometheus Group: Secaucus, NJ, Nov 3-5 2006.

Wallace, Kathe and Holly Herman. (2007). *Female Pelvic Floor: Function, Dysfunction and Treatment. Level 3.* The Prometheus Group: New York, NY, May 4-6 2007.

Wallace, Kathe and Holly Herman. (2008). *Female Pelvic Floor: Function, Dysfunction and Treatment. Level 1.* The Prometheus Group: Hunter College, March 7-9 2008.

Weiss, J. (2000). Chronic pelvic pain and myofascial trigger points. *The Pain Clinic,* 13(6), 13-18.

Weiss, J. (2001). Pelvic floor myofascial trigger point: Manual therapy for interstitial cystitis and the urgency-frequency syndrome. *The Journal of Urology,* 166(6), 2226-2231.

Weiss, J. (2003). Pudendal nerve entrapment. Presented at the *International Pelvic Pain Society 10th Scientific Meeting of Chronic Pelvic Pain* in Alberta, Canada August 2003, 1-25.

Wetzler, Gail, PT. (2009). *Gynecologic Visceral Manipulation.* Alexandria, VA: American Physical Therapy Association.

Wise, D. & Anderson, R. (2003). *A Headache in the Pelvis: A New Understanding and Treatment for Chronic Pelvic Pain Syndromes.* Occidental, CA: National Center for Pelvic Pain.

Wong CL, Lai KY, Tse HM. (2010). Effects of SP6 acupressure on pain and menstrual distress in young women with dysmenorrhea. *Complement Ther Clin Pract.* May;16(2):64-9. Epub 2009 Nov 14.

Appendix 1: Relevant Female Anatomy Diagrams

Use these diagrams of **Anterior and Posterior Female Muscles** to become familiar with the muscles in the body. This will help you with the exercises, tools and techniques in this book.

Anterior Female Muscles

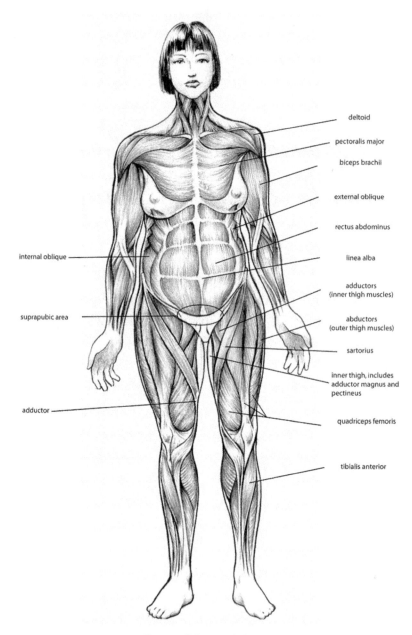

deltoid

pectoralis major

biceps brachii

external oblique

rectus abdominus

internal oblique

linea alba

adductors
(inner thigh muscles)

suprapubic area

abductors
(outer thigh muscles)

sartorius

inner thigh, includes
adductor magnus and
pectineus

adductor

quadriceps femoris

tibialis anterior

Source: Winston Johnson

Posterior Female Muscles

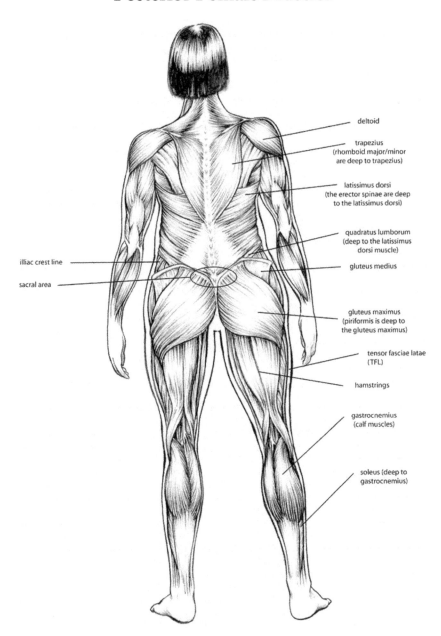

deltoid

trapezius
(rhomboid major/minor
are deep to trapezius)

latissimus dorsi
(the erector spinae are deep
to the latissimus dorsi)

quadratus lumborum
(deep to the latissimus
dorsi muscle)

gluteus medius

illiac crest line

sacral area

gluteus maximus
(piriformis is deep to
the gluteus maximus)

tensor fasciae latae
(TFL)

hamstrings

gastrocnemius
(calf muscles)

soleus (deep to
gastrocnemius)

Source: Winston Johnson

Appendix 2: Resources

www.PelvicPainRelief.com:
State-of-the-art online education and resources,
created by author Isa Herrera, MSPT, CSCS.

Additional Resources:

American College of Obstetricians and Gynecologists. Resource
Guide *www.acog.org.*

American Physical Therapy Association. 1-800-999-APTA. Physical
Therapy for the pelvic floor- Select Women's Health.
www.APTA.org.

The Business of Being Born. Great information for all women
planning to have a baby. *www.thebusinessofbeingborn.com.*

Dilator Sets. Available on this site. *www.vaginismus.com.*

Doulas of North America. It is our philosophy that all women should
have a doula for prenatal and postpartum care. *www.dona.org/*

Endometriosis Association. *www.endometriosisassn.org.*

Health Organization for Pudendal Education. *www.PudendalHope.info*

Herbal and Flower Products. For herbal and flower remedies *www.mountainroseherbs.com.*

Holly Herman & Kathe Wallace. Best teachers in pelvic floor rehab. Call to get a recommendation for a pelvic floor rehab specialist: 1- 646-355-8777. *http://hermanwallace.com.*

Interstitial Cystitis Network. *www.IC-network.org.*

Interstitial Cystitis Association. *www.IChelp.org.*

International Cesarean Awareness Network. *www.ICAN-online.org.*

International Society for the Study of Vulvovaginal Disease. *www.issvd.org.*

IPPS: The International Pelvic Pain Society. *www.PelvicPain.org.*

Kelly Brogan, MD. Holistic psychiatrist with tons of great information on post-partum depression and a great blog. *www.kellybroganMD.com.*

Midwives Alliance of North America. *www.mana.org.*

My Best Birth. Ricki Lake and Abby Epstein's great resource for women. *www. mybestbirth.com.*

National Fibromyalgia Association. *www.fmaware.org.*

NVA: National Vulvodynia Association. *www.NVA.org.*

Penny Simkin. The original pioneer physical therapist for childbirth education and labor support. *www.PennySimkin.com*

Pudendal Neuralgia Association, Inc. *www.pudendalassociation.org*

Vulvodynia Online Resource. *www.vulvodynia.com.*

Young Living Essential Oils: *www.youngliving.com/en_US/.* For medical/therapeutic grade essential oils, shop at Young Living. This is the brand I trust the most. Please use my subscriber number ID #1422496 to get a wholesale membership. There is a small membership enrollment fee to buy oils at wholesale that ranges from $40 to $275.

Index

chakra, 21, 33, 38, 181, 228, 255-260, 274-278, 280, 282-286, 290, 292, 312, 325, 335

chi, 28, 103, 255-256, 259, 288-289, 293

childbirth, 38, 55, 59, 63, 68-70, 84-85, 93, 180, 296, 316, 319, 327, 332, 346

Chlamydia, 92

chlorinated, 68, 71

Chronic, 32, 42, 93, 296-297, 312, 325, 328, 330, 333, 335, 339-340

Circulation, 28, 30-31, 64, 75, 102, 135

clitoris, 44-49, 52, 58, 62-63, 93, 105, 188, 221, 266, 275, 319

clock, 49, 56-60, 63, 185, 218, 221-222, 224, 260, 275-276

Coccygeus, 186

Coccygodynia, 312, 335

collagen, 66

colloidal, 69

Conception, 29, 33, 37-38, 40, 100

congestion, 34, 39, 75, 103, 155, 255

Connection, 33, 37-38, 42, 97, 102-103, 146, 196, 200, 209, 259, 276, 322

Connective, 94, 119, 126, 181, 228, 231, 260, 269-270, 311-313, 316-317, 320-321

Constipation, 68, 75, 81, 123, 181, 296-297, 299

continence, 80, 179, 204, 209, 211, 215, 217, 327

Contraction, 30, 33, 35, 87, 105, 118, 137-138, 148, 155-156, 159, 164, 168, 171, 174, 187-190, 197, 201, 203, 205, 229, 238-239, 241, 300, 305-306, 315-317, 337

contraindications, 308

Coordination, 98, 187, 191, 193, 199, 205-206

core, 21, 114, 119, 135, 137, 159, 205, 224, 227-232, 236, 239-241, 250, 282, 296, 307

corrective techniques, 156

cramps, 34, 141, 167, 169, 181

cranberry, 89, 106

crunches, 21, 227-228, 235, 297

Cyctocele, 307

Cystitis, 83, 89, 329, 336, 339, 346

cysts, 75

defecation, 68, 70, 81, 118, 121, 123, 148, 181, 297, 299, 315, 317

Diabetes, 323

diaphragm, 186, 193, 333, 339

Diastasis, 21, 119-120, 134, 228-231, 235, 239, 282, 296, 299, 313, 320

Diflucan, 69

dilator, 86, 88, 195, 261, 345

Dimples, 152, 318

Disc, 31, 120, 125-131, 147, 170, 297, 311, 314, 316

discharge, 63, 92, 308

discomfort, 72, 79, 138, 215, 277, 291, 307, 315, 323

disconnected, 43, 46, 256, 259, 276

discs, 126, 128-131

disease, 83-84, 91-92, 259, 308, 333, 346

Donut, 126, 128, 314

douches, 68

doula, 86, 345

downtraining, 180, 192, 195

DRA, 21, 119-120, 137, 231-238, 240, 252, 296

Dyna, 203-204, 238

dysfunction, 17, 19-21, 27-28, 50, 54, 61, 67, 83-86, 91, 93-94, 98-99, 103, 117, 120, 124, 135, 137, 141, 145, 147, 149, 158, 160-161, 164-165, 167, 170, 176-177, 180-182, 227-229, 231, 255, 297-298, 315, 317, 322, 328-329, 334, 336, 339

dyspareunia, 83, 90, 296, 334, 338

emotional, 29, 61, 81, 277, 335

endometriosis, 83, 90-91, 346

endorphin, 74

endurance, 135, 141, 179, 187, 189, 191, 197, 199-200, 205

energetic, 19, 29, 80, 227, 256, 277

episiotomy, 38, 54-55, 63, 70, 85, 91, 297, 313

epithelium, 90

Epsom, 69

erectile, 51

erogenous, 44, 102

erotic, 61, 177, 179, 225

Erythema, 86

Estriol, 71

estrogen, 296-297, 334

exam, 28, 44-45, 54, 80, 83, 86, 187-188, 316

examination, 43-45, 54, 63, 86, 187

exhalation, 193, 195, 317, 323

extremities, 191, 312, 318, 321

fascia, 79, 93, 97, 181, 228, 261, 311, 313, 321-322

fascial, 200, 228, 321

fatigue, 42, 88

fecal, 85, 183, 231, 296, 298, 318, 337

feet, 55, 122, 130-131, 150, 163, 168, 171, 174, 201, 203, 211, 236, 244,

250, 265, 267, 275, 279, 281, 285, 287-288, 305-306, 316

fertility, 40, 75, 103, 330

fiber, 68, 87, 123, 190, 223, 319

fibroids, 75, 83

fibromyalgia, 88, 346

Fibrosus, 311, 314-315

fibrosus, 311, 314-315

fibrous, 91, 231

flatulence, 215, 217

flexed, 122, 208, 316

flexor, 172, 175, 314

foods, 89, 106-108, 114

forceps, 85, 297

genital, 37, 92-93, 333

girdle, 142, 144-148, 156-158, 317

gland, 45-46, 48, 62, 257, 289-290

gluteal, 74, 81, 88, 106, 169, 183, 204, 211, 213, 302-303, 312-313, 321-322

gratitude, 289-291, 293

groin, 120, 128, 147, 161, 174, 320

gynecological, 28, 33, 36, 85-86, 91, 93, 325

gynecologist, 60-61, 63, 84, 179, 345

herb, 64-66, 108

herbal, 108, 346

Herniation, 126-127, 284

hips, 69, 73, 88-89, 103, 122, 126-127, 130-131, 150, 158-159, 163, 207, 209, 213, 215-216, 228, 236, 238, 245, 248, 251, 264, 267, 279, 281, 299, 301-302, 311, 316

holes, 321

holistic, 19, 75, 114, 346

hormones, 61, 87, 314

hymenectomy, 91

hypertonic, 50, 180

hypotonic, 180

Hysterectomy, 91, 93, 296-297, 307

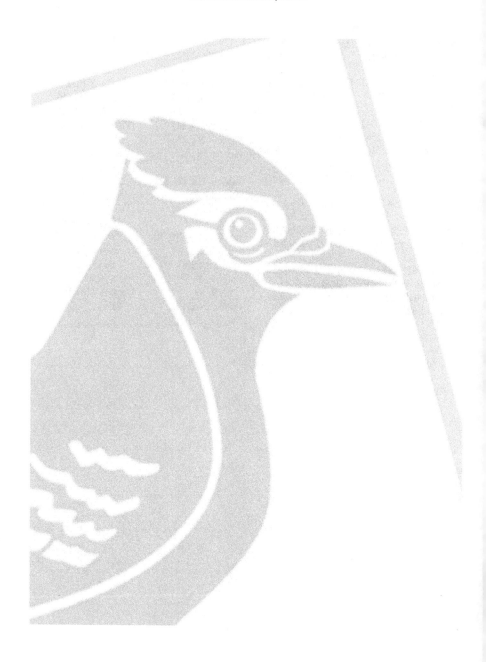